Praise for *The*

"A thoughtful, patient, ultimately fasc... nineteenth-century science, and society, to come to grips with the germ theory of illness, and develop new technologies to take on one of humanity's oldest scourges, tuberculosis." —*Forbes*

"*The Remedy* is a highly entertaining, interesting, and thought-provoking book, leaving the reader with a much deeper appreciation of how much safer—and in many ways, predictable—our lives are today thanks to the toil and efforts of men such as Robert Koch and his contemporaries." —*The Boston Globe*

"Goetz's passion for his subject and quick-witted intellectual engagement renders *The Remedy* immensely pleasurable." —*The Lancet*

"A gripping story . . . with great verve, painting word pictures full of color and telling detail . . . vividly evokes the rivalries rife in the scientific world." —*The Washington Times*

"An enjoyable chronicle." —*The Wall Street Journal*

"Weaves the suspense of a Sherlock Holmes mystery into a tale of ambition, obsession, scientific discovery, and skepticism at the dawn of modern medicine." —*Discover*

"Goetz weaves together a compelling narrative, chronicling the struggle to find the causes and cures for some of the most ferocious diseases that have stalked humans (and animals) through time: cholera, smallpox, anthrax, and tuberculosis. . . . Perhaps most importantly, *The Remedy* reminds us of how far we have come, and how much we take for granted in modern medicine." —*BookPage*

"*The Remedy* achieves a rare feat: serious, accurate scientific writing that is also engaging and entertaining." —*Shelf Awareness*

"An intriguing medical and literary history . . . fascinating, convergent stories [of] doggedly inquisitive men who discovered that neither germs nor crime are any match for science." —*Publishers Weekly*

"A beguiling real-life medical detective story." —*Kirkus Reviews*

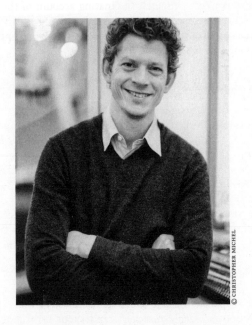

Thomas Goetz is a science journalist and health-care innovator. The entrepreneur-in-residence at the Robert Wood Johnson Foundation, he is also cofounder of the health technology company Iodine. The former executive editor of *Wired*, his writing has been selected for *The Best American Science Writing* and *The Best Technology Writing* anthologies. He holds a master of public health degree from the University of California, Berkeley, and a master's in literature from the University of Virginia. He lives in San Francisco with his wife and two boys.

CONNECT ONLINE
───────────────
www.thomasgoetz.com
twitter.com/tgoetz

THE
REMEDY

ROBERT KOCH,

ARTHUR CONAN DOYLE, AND

THE QUEST TO CURE TUBERCULOSIS

THOMAS GOETZ

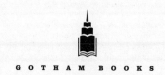

GOTHAM BOOKS

GOTHAM BOOKS
Published by the Penguin Group
Penguin Group (USA) LLC
375 Hudson Street
New York, New York 10014

USA | Canada | UK | Ireland | Australia | New Zealand | India | South Africa | China
penguin.com
A Penguin Random House Company

Previously published as a Gotham Books hardcover

First trade paperback printing, March 2015

1   3   5   7   9   10   8   6   4   2

Gotham Books and the skyscraper logo are trademarks of Penguin Group (USA) LLC

The Library of Congress has catalogued the hardcover edition of this book as follows:
Goetz, Thomas, 1968 November 14– author.
The remedy : Robert Koch, Arthur Conan Doyle, and the quest to cure
tuberculosis / Thomas Goetz.
p. ; cm.
Includes bibliographical references and index.
ISBN 978-1-592-40751-4 (HC)   978-1-592-40917-4 (PBK)
I. Title.
[DNLM: 1. Doyle, Arthur Conan, 1859–1930. 2. Koch, Robert, 1843–1910. 3. Tuberculosis—history—Europe. 4. Tuberculosis—history—United States. 5. Germ Theory of Disease—history—Europe. 6. Germ Theory of Disease—history—United States. 7. History, 18th Century—Europe. 8. History, 18th Century—United States. 9. History, 19th Century—Europe. 10. History, 19th Century—United States. WF 11 GA1]
RA644.T7
614.5'42—dc23   2013039611

Illustration on page ix from *Review of Reviews, 1890*. Photograph on page 3 courtesy of Humboldt University of Berlin, University Archives. Photographs on pages 25 and 85 courtesy of Robert Koch Institute. Photograph on page 53 by Felix Nadar. Photographs on pages 111 and 139 courtesy of University of Minnesota Libraries. Photograph on page 161 by the author. Photograph on page 189 by Bain News Service, image courtesy of Library of Congress. Illustration on page 211 by Sidney Paget. Image on page 227 courtesy of the National Library of Medicine. Image on page 245 courtesy of National Museum of American History (photographer unknown).

Printed in the United States of America
Set in Adobe Caslon   •   Designed by Elke Sigal

In memory of Frederick C. Goetz and Cecilia M. Goetz

CONTENTS

The Disease

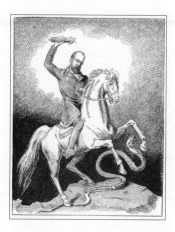

Robert Koch, as depicted at the height of his fame, 1890

In train after train, consumptives filled the passenger cars, their hacks and coughs competing with steam whistles and screaming brakes as the engines came to a halt in Potsdamer Platz. They came to Berlin without any sense of where to go or what to do once they arrived. And they kept coming, for days, weeks, and months. It must have struck Berliners as a sort of zombie pilgrimage: Here were the walking dead of Europe, all suddenly flocking to their city in search of *something*—some fantastic substance that did not yet officially exist.

They began arriving in August 1890, when rumors first began to circulate that a treatment, a *remedy*, for consumption, or tuberculosis, had been discovered by Europe's greatest scientist, Robert Koch. Koch made no promises; he had only hinted at a substance that seemed to arrest the disease. But a hint was all it took. This was the deadliest disease in the world, and these were the most desperate souls. If there was hope to be had in Berlin, they would seek it out.

Tuberculosis was a cunning disease, coming on slowly, almost casually. At first it seemed innocuous, beginning with a cough; a cold, perhaps, or a touch of bad air. But then that cough turned malevolent, becoming stronger and more painful and extracting blood with each spasm. Then the appetite would go, replaced by fatigue, a deep dullness that would pull the sufferers into lethargy. Eventually, bodies would begin to wither and dissipate from within. For most consumptives, this played out over months and years. Even when the end seemed imminent, it was as if the consumptives could not muster the energy to die—until, finally, they did, by the thousands and hundreds of thousands and millions. In the last half of the nineteenth century, at least one-quarter of all deaths were due to tuberculosis, a steady pall that loomed over every country in Europe, over the United States, and indeed worldwide.

So the consumptives came to Berlin, and inevitably, death came with them. They died in the passenger cars on the way to the city, they died in the hotels, and they died in the clinics and hospitals where they waited for a dose of this extraordinary remedy. The city didn't know what to do with them all. Hotels and hospitals filled up. Coffeehouses were converted into sanitariums.

With concern rising that Berlin's own population was at an increased risk of infection, the Berlin police department began instituting emergency measures to control the onslaught. Joseph Lister himself, one of the most famous physicians in Europe and a pioneer of the germ theory of disease, suggested that the horde created a "serious danger to the public health of this city likely to arise from the sudden invasion of patients suffering from every form of tuberculosis and coming from all the corners of the earth."

The tide grew still larger after November 13, when Koch finally offered some specifics for his remedy. A public demonstration of the substance was scheduled for November 17 in Berlin, and now scientists crowded among the consumptives on the trains. The finest medical men in Europe were all eager to see firsthand how Koch's substance could destroy the worst disease humanity had ever known.

On one of those trains was a young Scottish physician, making the pilgrimage not for the cure, but to scrutinize the evidence behind it. This man, an unknown provincial doctor who yearned to become something greater, was en route to play detective and to assess what Dr. Koch had created. He idolized Koch, but his years in practice had hardened him to the promise of quick cures and easy fixes. He was headed to Berlin to discern whether this remedy might really work. And this trip would change his life: He would arrive as an observer of history but leave as a figure in it. He would arrive as a physician but leave as a writer.

This doctor's name was Arthur Conan Doyle.

DEADLY AS IT WAS, HORRIBLE AS IT WAS, TUBERCULOSIS WAS ALSO entirely ordinary in the last decades of the nineteenth century. For that entire century, the numbers are staggering. In England, as many as a quarter of all deaths were due to consumption. In the United States, the disease was the leading cause of death; in German towns, tuberculosis was the second-largest killer, after gastrointestinal diseases—but when one includes deaths attributed to generic "lung" conditions, most of which are likely to have been TB, it accounts for a plurality of deaths by far.

These figures are fuzzy and, if anything, probably underestimated the scope of the disease. Record keeping was poor at the time, and tuberculosis often traveled under aliases. Manifest in the lungs, it was known as consumption or phthisis; on the skin, it was called scrofula or lupus; it could also appear in other organs and be mistaken for cancer. It wreaked most of its toll in its pulmonary form, and it couldn't have chosen a better hiding place. Deep inside the lungs, tuberculosis could take so long to make its creep that, for many, death seemed to come from some other cause—influenza or pneumonia or some fever—leaving the true underlying disease invisible, a shadow in the background.

Not that anybody—even public officials, even family—was all that concerned about the precise cause of death in general in the mid- to late nineteenth century. After all, these were the hours just before the dawn of modern medicine, when neither diagnosis (such as it was) nor treatment (such as it was) could be of much use. When death could come from any direction for any reason at any time, questions about cause didn't seem so important. Fathers, mothers, husbands, wives, children, siblings—whatever took them, they were gone, like so many others.

Indeed, it is difficult to imagine, from the security of our twenty-first-century perspective, how familiar death was in the late nineteenth century. Suffering, injury, and disease were altogether routine, part of the ordinary experience of everyday life. People tend to use average life span to illustrate historic differences in health, but those figures—in 1870 the average life span in Europe and the United States was about thirty-six years, compared to about eighty years today—don't nearly make the point strongly enough. Rather, to get a true sense of the pervasiveness of death, one must look at the annual death rate: how many of the living ended up dead every year.

In England circa 1870, twenty-two people out of a thousand died every year. This means that more than 2 percent of the population was dying off every year, a constant deduction in humanity and accretion of misery. Today, the death rate is about five per one thousand, which is to say, *four times* as many people were dying then than are now.

Today, we just can't conceive of so much death, all the time, all around us. Death is so unfamiliar today that almost any expiration seems exceptional. We lament the passing of the generations as if each loss were a tragedy rather than biology. But in 1870, death was a constant presence, lurking around every corner, something that visited families and friends regularly (if not routinely). The dead came from all stages of life: the old, of course, but also those in the prime of life. Back then, every year, nearly 2 percent of those between ages thirty-five and forty-four died, and those between forty-five and fifty-four died at twice that rate. And then there were the very young. Infant mortality in England and the United States hovered around a stunning 20 percent of all live births—and in some areas, a rate of 30 to 40 percent wasn't uncommon. (Today, the infant mortality rate is about four per one thousand live births, twenty times less than it was in 1870.) And though wealth offered some protection, this carnage largely knew no class boundaries, afflicting the rich and the poor alike.

The causes were inadequately tabulated and even less understood, but the categories were as common to the nineteenth century as they are obscure to us today. There were the deadly fevers (scarlet fever, spotted fever, puerperal fever, typhoid fever) that made every spike in temperature fearful. Once or twice a year, pneumonia and influenza would sweep through a community, culling the weak, the old, the young. There were outbreaks of cholera; not the stomach flu of today, this was a horrid bout of diarrhea and vomiting that would slaughter whole families in a fortnight and then move on to take the neighbors as well. And if disease wasn't bad enough, there were the many accidents and their consequences, the trauma of a broken bone or a deep cut often leading to infection, gangrene, and death. (Twice as many people died from accidents in 1870 as they do today.)

And most of all, there was consumption. In nineteenth-century Europe and the United States, this was the most common of all ways to die. It was a languid, almost casual disease, the first chronic disease, in many respects. As a result, few doctors believed that there could be anything contagious about it whatsoever. Rather, it seemed largely hereditary, passed along in families with "weak constitutions."

As for treatments, there was no end of them: tonics and salves and cod-liver oil. These were hardly cures; at best, they seemed restorative. But, as one pamphlet warned, "To the drowning man, a stick, a straw, or any old piece of wood looks like a help to save himself from death. So, to the consumptive, any kind of flimsy statement or any brand of manufactured 'patent' medicine appears to offer a hope of cure and a chance for life."

In truth, there was no true remedy for tuberculosis, no drug that would dispatch the disease and restore the individual. Some doctors despaired that there would ever be a cure for it and felt that any offer of treatment was deceitful and unethical. They chose to treat it not as a disease but, rather, as a fact of life, counseling patients to learn to live with the condition as long as they might. Instead of scrounging for a cure, they should reconcile themselves to the fact that their fate had been determined. Whether brought on by God or family, consumption was their lot.

In fact, tuberculosis is caused by a microbe particularly suited to humans (and, curiously, to cows). This bacteria, *Mycobacterium tuberculosis,* seems almost engineered to exploit the human tendency to mask fear with denial: It is perfectly content to spend years in the human body, making itself inconspicuous as the infection slowly spreads, until it at last reveals itself to its human host. But in 1870 it was not only invisible; it was inconceivable. There was no way to fathom that a disease such as consumption could be the work of a contagion, a germ. The very notion of germs was radical, an idea outside the bounds of traditional medicine. *Perhaps* diseases such as smallpox or measles—which came on quickly, appeared to spread from person to person, and produced symptoms visible to the naked eye—had some contagion behind them. But consumption bore none of those characteristics.

Still, some scientists had started to investigate the idea that tiny "animalcules," as they were described, invisible to the human eye, might be agents of disease. In France, Louis Pasteur had done the most to advance such notions, and since at least 1850 this idea, referred to as "the germ theory," had been much discussed in Europe. Using microscopes (which, like the stethoscope, had only recently been widely adopted by medical science), some had begun to identify tiny particles in the blood, chains of cells that seemed to move and grow and even reproduce. To those who believed in the germ theory, the vision of these microbes opened the door to a new era of science and a new utility to medicine. Dr. John Tyndall, one of England's most prominent scientists and essayists, was among these believers; in a lecture entitled "On Haze and Dust," delivered before the Royal Institution of Great Britain in January 1870, he thrilled to the idea. "When he clearly eyes his quarry, the eagle's strength is doubled, and his swoop is rendered sure," he told his colleagues. "If the germ theory be proved true it will give a definiteness to our efforts to stamp out disease which they could not previously possess."

Tyndall's argument was dynamic, enthusiastic—and tentative. As his hedging made clear, with its "*if* the germ theory be proved true" caveat, the theory was still largely conjecture. There was no certainty to it, no evidence that these curious organisms under the microscope had any real relation to disease. For a matter of science, this was a mortal deficiency. Lacking proof, the germ theory would drift outside the harbors of science, an alluring idea, but one unmoored to the day-to-day reality of medicine.

PICTURE, IF YOU WILL, THE PROVERBIAL DOCTOR'S BAG, A LEATHER satchel filled with the tools of the modern general practitioner: antibiotics; aspirin; a stethoscope, otoscope, and various other scopes; a blood pressure monitor; a prescription pad. Now open the bag and turn it upside down, shaking loose all those implements that didn't exist in 1870. Though one or two tools might remain—the stethoscope or the speculum—the bag would be mostly empty. In fact, most of the resources that constitute modern medicine had not arrived by 1870, and those ideas and instruments that did exist were novel, regarded by many as avant-garde gadgets that threatened a doctor's autonomy.

This isn't to say that the last quarter of the nineteenth century was the Dark Ages of medicine; rather, it was when the light started to break. After two millennia of misapprehension, medicine was finally shaking off its attachment to the "four humors" (blood, phlegm, and black and yellow bile) and turning to the more empirical disciplines of pathology and microscopy. In 1858 the first edition of *Gray's Anatomy* appeared, giving clear, accurate illustrations of the human body. In the 1850s and '60s, medical laboratories began to appear in Europe and the United States, separate from hospitals and doctors' offices, designed as distinct quarters for scientific inquiry and discovery. Surgery was just emerging as a respectable trade, recently delivered from the era of hacksaws and slugs of whiskey by the discovery of reliable anesthetics. "Gentlemen, this is no humbug," remarked one witness to a demonstration of ether at the Massachusetts General Hospital in 1846. Within a decade, surgery was a booming trade and, increasingly, a respectable one as well.

But for those physicians tasked with caring for patients, their bags remained discouragingly bare. Practically speaking, not much really worked. For prevention, there was a smallpox vaccine (developed in 1796 by Edward Jenner but made compulsory in Britain only in the 1850s and '60s), but little else. For treatment, there were salves and ointments and tonics, but almost nothing that we would today consider a real, functional medication. For every opiate or digitalis (an extract of the foxglove plant that was used to treat dropsy, or heart failure), there were cabinets of cod-liver oil and other elixirs, the best of which were harmless, the worst of which were outright poisons. In short, medicine had very little to offer in the way of effective treatments that would truly heal or cure.

On the other hand, public health—which focuses on the populace's well-being (in contrast to clinical medicine's concern with individual cases)—had made more headway by 1870, with ideas such as hygiene and sanitation finding allies in municipal governments. After decades of increasingly virulent cholera outbreaks, the largest cities in Europe (London, Paris, Berlin, and Naples) began massive sewer projects in the 1850s and '60s. These were constructed under the as-sumption that disease came from the smell emanating from the waste, not the germs the waste contained, but the result was the same: cleaner cities and improved health. Even so, these ideas were just emerging, and the most basic measures of public health—starting with the idea of just counting who died of what—were controversial, seen by medical doctors as challenging their authority and their duties to individual patients.

Then, like so much else in these waning years of the 1800s, things began to change.

THE LAST DECADES OF THE NINETEENTH CENTURY WERE REPLETE with new discoveries. A list of inventions from 1875 to 1900 serves as nothing less than an inventory of the toolbox for modern life: the telephone, the lightbulb, the phonograph, the fountain pen, the cash register, the dishwasher, the escalator, the vacuum cleaner, the modern bicycle, the internal combustion engine, the Kodak camera, the flashbulb, the X-ray machine, the radio, the tape recorder, the paper clip, the zipper, subways, electric power plants, and drinking straws. All these modern tools were invented in a burst of innovation unprecedented in human history.

Significantly, these were improvements at the human scale. Each of these inventions (even drinking straws) came with the promise of making life's daily toils a little less complicated and a little more comfortable. They offered an irresistible step into the future, when things wouldn't be *quite so much work.* "If once tried," promised an advertisement for one of the most marvelous of all the era's discoveries, "this will always afterwards be used." The great invention in this case was perforated toilet paper, but the description could apply equally to most of the tools and products that transformed the lives of everyday people.

Though it was hardly apparent (or even relevant) to the average consumer, all these discoveries were the consequence of the scientific and engineering breakthroughs from earlier in the century. The X-ray machine was the result of Wilhelm Roentgen's work on electromagnetic radiation; the gasoline-powered engine required a new understanding of chemistry; the electrical inventions were the fruit of Michael Faraday's work on electromagnetism and electrochemistry in the 1820s and '30s; even the classic Gem paper clip would have been impossible before discoveries in both chemistry and electricity allowed steel to be galvanized. All these inventions were born of science that had happened just a few years earlier.

Medical science, though, lagged behind. The breakthroughs that would inform modern medicine had yet to appear by 1870. But over the next quarter century, those insights would come, and medicine would begin to scratch at the big mysteries of life and death and illness. Vaccines and antitoxins and medications began to suggest a way not just to understand these mysteries, but also perhaps to solve them, to remedy them.

And so here is our story: In August 1891 two men of science crossed paths in Berlin in what would be an episode of historic magnitude. Their encounter would change the trajectory of each of their lives and begin to transform the course of science itself.

The first is Robert Koch, a medical doctor turned bacteriologist. Though today Koch's name is little known outside his native Germany or university microbiology departments, he was, in his day, the most celebrated scientist on earth. With a single-mindedness bordering on righteousness, he pursued the idea that many diseases are caused by germs and that those germs can be isolated and identified. Koch's great nemesis would be tuberculosis; it was the province of his greatest discovery and his most tragic disgrace.

Through a quirk of history, Koch's undoing was put in motion by another physician: Arthur Conan Doyle. Conan Doyle is famous to us today as the creator of Sherlock Holmes, but his brush with Koch took place while he was still a practicing doctor in England; literature was then only a diversion. Like Koch, Conan Doyle saw the world through a scientific lens, one that informed his medical career and also, quite profoundly, his stories. It's not too much to say that, without Robert Koch, and without this encounter, there may never have been a Sherlock Holmes as we know him.

For years, Koch and Conan Doyle's story has merited at most a curious footnote, a coincidental intersection of two dissimilar biographies. But in truth, theirs was a historic if unwitting collaboration. Koch and Conan Doyle shared more than a passing coincidence; they shared a trajectory from the nineteenth century of leeches and cod-liver oil to the twentieth century of microscopes and antibiotics. Though circumstances placed these men at odds, history might now consider them comrades, joined in a battle for science over superstition, for process over haste, for scrutiny over supposition, for data over dogma. What Koch accomplished in the laboratory, Conan Doyle appropriated in his literature. What Koch proved to science, Conan Doyle proved to society. And, ultimately, both their lives would be undone by tuberculosis.

This book also tells a larger tale about how medicine became modern and where cures come from. And it helps us answer some larger questions: How does a scorned idea grow to acceptance and then revolution? And what does it mean to cure a disease, to ward off death so that many millions of people can live?

If there's one caution to this tale, it's this: Avoid the temptation to read the story, and the science within it, as the inevitable march of progress, a predetermined direction for human history. Especially where scientific investigations are concerned, it's a fallacy to treat history as an unstoppable trajectory away from ignorance and toward insight. Though we can, retrospectively, catalog science along a tidy arc from one discovery to another, the actual course of research is

THE
REMEDY

PART I

CHAPTER I

1871 · The Doctor in Wöllstein

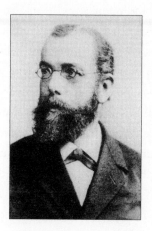

Photo of Robert Koch, circa 1882

On January 16, 1871, in the French city of Orléans, Robert Koch was exactly where he'd hoped to be: in a field hospital, up to his elbows in the blood and pus and piss of war. The hospital, such as it was, was a converted train station in the center of town. In the distance, from more than a hundred kilometers away, came the boom of cannons, the German artillery shelling French troops in the Siege of Paris.

When the young doctor first applied to join the German effort against the French, the previous July, he was rejected on account of his nearsightedness. But a few months later, Koch tenaciously applied a second time. By now, the growing scope of the war had lowered the bar to entry, and he was accepted. Koch was assigned to the medical unit, given some rudimentary instructions on trauma surgery and care, and dispatched to a field hospital a mile or two behind the front lines. After a couple of movements, he was now in Orléans, with a battle raging a few kilometers outside of town. Litters of soldiers, their bodies torn to pieces, were being carried to the makeshift medical facility.

"The situation of the wounded or ill soldiers is mostly different from what the public thinks about it," he wrote to his parents. "I was sadly eyewitness to scenes that prove that a human life is worth nothing, even though they might be saved with a little effort. Every romanticism that people project into the war who know the war from books is nothing against the uncountable bad experiences that you encounter as participant in a war." At twenty-seven years old, Robert Koch was finally getting the dose of adventure he had craved—and it was more brutal than he could ever have imagined.

At five and a half feet tall with a slight build, a soft chin, and a stern face, Koch was hardly imposing. He was socially tentative and had a thin, high voice. Heretofore, little in his life had been exceptional, and there was little reason to believe that would change once the war ended.

But while it lasted, the war gave Koch a purpose. In the field hospital he worked on a dozen men at once; he would rush from one desperate case to another with scarcely time to wipe the muck off his hands. Some soldiers, their limbs barely attached, needed an immediate amputation. Others required some bandages and a few hours' rest on a cot before being sent back into the battle. And some could only be covered with blankets stiff with the blood of their comrades so that they might die with at least a modicum of comfort.

The son of an engineer, Koch was born in December 1843 in Clausthal, a small mining town in the Harz Mountains, in central Germany. One of thirteen children, eight of them sons, Koch grew up yearning for some sort of adventure in life, to break out of the middle. He began his studies hoping to be a naturalist, at the time the most glamorous of the sciences. The nineteenth century had begun with the explorations of Alexander von Humboldt, the Prussian naturalist who won worldwide fame studying the climate and geology of Latin America. In the 1830s, Charles Darwin embarked on his voyages on the HMS *Beagle,* publishing his observations on botany and biology to great renown. In 1859 he published his *On the Origin of Species,* making science seem at once revolutionary and relevant. These scientists lived lives of romance and adventure, and they inspired young Koch. The natural sciences promised opportunity. Every expedition seemed to yield great progress, tremendous leaps forward in human knowledge.

But dreams were one thing, and the realities of the Koch family were another: Robert watched with envy as two older brothers emigrated to the United States. Then he enrolled at Göttingen University, where he would study that most prosaic and tenuous of sciences—medicine. Göttingen was surely chosen out of convenience: It was just fifty kilometers down the road from Clausthal. But it was more than just a provincial school. Unlike France, where Paris was the absolute center of science and academic research, Germany was a decentralized nation. The German state was not officially unified until 1871, when Otto von Bismarck consolidated the German peoples into one nation. Germany had thus developed a network of intellectual centers, in Berlin and Munich, but likewise in Heidelberg, Wittenberg, Halle, Göttingen, and other cities. In the 1860s, when Koch attended university, science was flourishing throughout the country, from Breslau in the east to Heidelberg in the west and Munich in the south. Göttingen University was a thriving center of physical sciences, a hub of new ideas in biology and medicine. There, Koch had the opportunity to study with Georg Meissner, a master scientist and an innovator in devising animal experiments, and Friedrich Henle, a pioneer in microscopy.

In the late 1840s and early 1850s, Henle had published his *Handbook of Rational Pathology,* which made an early case that living agents—he called them contagions—could cause human disease. "The contagion is not itself the disease, but the *inducer* of the disease," Henle wrote. "If it could be possible to prove that a contagion can be cultured outside the body . . . then such a contagion could only be a plant or an animal." *If it could be possible to prove*—Henle wanted to pinpoint microbes as the cause of disease, but he could only gesture at the proof; he could not provide it.

Henle was a good match for Koch, as both were chronically shy, more inclined to heads-down research than to socializing. From Henle, Koch learned the techniques of a master microscopist: a great attention to detail, thoroughness, and care of process. As it happened, Koch was at Göttingen while Henle was hard at work on his magnum opus, a three-volume assessment of human anatomy titled the *Handbook of Systematic Human Anatomy*. (The first volume was published in 1866, the year Koch graduated.) This was the first great work of anatomical description since Vesalius's historic *On the Structure of the Human Body* three centuries earlier. Where Vesalius's breakthrough was to make an unflinching assessment of human anatomy, teasing out the networks of organs and nerves and vessels in human flesh, Henle's innovation was to turn the microscope to the next order of magnitude, noting the structures within organs, the sheaths of cells around nerve fibers and ligaments, parsing the rods and cones within the human eye.

At twenty-two, in 1866, Koch passed the state medical examination and was tempted by his brothers' calls to join them in America. He briefly considered becoming a ship's doctor and seeing the world. Instead, he impetuously returned to Clausthal and married his hometown sweetheart, Emma Fraatz. Emma was the youngest daughter of an official of the local evangelical church, and Koch had kept company with her before leaving for Göttingen. She was a serious and practical young woman, and she quickly made clear that she would not be leaving Germany for some foreign adventure. Koch was in Germany to stay.

Koch first found a position at a local facility for disabled children in Langenhagen, a small village near Hanover. On the side, he set up a practice attending to the needs of the local villagers. He and Emma lived in a few rooms in the house of a local farmer. Soon enough his practice was flourishing, and he had enough money to buy a small carriage (a useful status symbol for the young doctor) and enough time to ramble through local marshes collecting various plants and water samples, which he'd bring home and examine under a cheap microscope. One evening, when he returned home from the clinic, Emma told him she was pregnant. Life for Robert Koch seemed to be settling in comfortably, if modestly.

But the calm was soon over. His institution had financial problems, and his position, he was informed, was being eliminated. Koch would have to make his way somewhere else. First he tried Braetz, but three months later he'd moved again to Niemegk, a village near Potsdam. The townspeople there seemed to prefer faith healers to physicians, though, and Koch struggled to find patients. Emma, now caring for their daughter, Gertrud, began to grow frustrated with Robert's efforts. "It's going awful here," she wrote to her father from Niemegk in 1869. "We have to skimp and save every penny and I'm still not sure we'll make it. I keep telling Robert we have to leave here, that he MUST find a better position, but Robert has given up all hope and now has the idea again to go overseas. He can't make up his mind about anything."

At last they moved again, to Rackwitz, a town then in eastern Prussia, now in Poland. The family took an apartment over the post office, and Koch got a few patients. Emma seemed more hopeful than she'd been in months. Things improved considerably after a local gentleman, the Baron von Unruhe-Bomst, shot himself with a revolver. Koch successfully treated him for the wound, and soon more patients were coming his way. He began to turn his little yard into a naturalist's laboratory, with pigeons, chickens, and a beehive. He even began going to the local beer hall with the town mayor. Once again, things seemed to be back on track for young Dr. Koch.

THEN, IN JULY 1870, THE WAR BEGAN. KOCH WATCHED THREE OF HIS seven brothers join the French War, as the Franco-Prussian War was called in Germany. For Koch, it was the chance to do *something*, to turn his safe but anonymous life toward something greater. Out there, in France, heroes were dying on battlefields; men were making their mark; history was being written. If he couldn't take his wife and new daughter to America, Koch decided to choose the path open to him. After scarcely consulting with Emma, he went to war.

He was first posted to a field hospital near Metz, the capital of the Lorraine region of France, where he slept in a hayloft. "The smell of dead bodies, many dead horses and thousands of bags, guns and helmets were near the rural road, at least this was what we could see in the darkness," he wrote to his father. "We drink a cup of black coffee, of course, without sugar or milk and eat a piece of dry bread. At noon there is boiled beef and bread again or maybe even a thin soup. . . . One has no appetite for a second plate," he wrote, though he did admit that the local wine was worth drinking.

At Metz, the Prussian army had tied up 180,000 French troops and 70,000 citizens in a months-long siege. With food running short and dysentery and cholera spreading, the French tried repeatedly to battle their way out of the city. Each time, they were pushed back by the Germans, with enough casualties among the Prussian troops to keep Koch and his fellows in the medical corps busy. For a fledgling doctor such as Koch, used to treating injured farmers and their pregnant wives, the tumult of the siege was a dizzying mix of duty, disgust, and opportunity. It gave him his first glimpse of the true mechanism of death: not the wound, but the infection that came later. Eventually the French began to starve, and they surrendered the city on October 27.

Koch was then transferred 120 kilometers to the south, to Neuf-château, a French town already occupied by the Prussians. There he was stationed at a hospital for soldiers suffering from typhoid fever. Today we understand typhoid to be an infectious disease caused by the *Salmonella* bacterium and typically spread through exposure to feces or similar unsanitary conditions. But in 1870 it was little understood, perhaps contagious, perhaps spread through tainted water. Generally, it was simply considered one of the risks of war. At the hospital, Koch had his hands full; the Germans suffered more than 73,000 cases of typhoid during the war, with nearly 9,000 fatalities.

Koch's experience with typhoid was eye-opening. After the initial fever, the infection settles in the intestines, inflaming the organs and distending the abdomen. As it spreads to other organs—the pancreas, the liver—internal bleeding becomes likely, resulting in bloody stool. Delirium is common, especially if the infection makes its way to the brain. The death rate in Koch's day was about 20 percent. Koch, who'd gotten a sense of the microbial world from Henle, must have suspected there was some agent at work, some unseen contagion spreading from soldier to soldier. But with no diagnostic tools or effective medicines, he could only watch, offering the comfort of a damp cloth or a blanket, as the sickness set in. It was depressing and hopeless work, and Koch despaired. He pined for simple things: a newspaper, a lamp, home-cooked food, his family. He must have been relieved when he was transferred once again, this time to the field hospital in Orléans.

At this point, Koch had been at war for nearly five months. The adventure was far messier than he'd anticipated. There were the sights—the severed limbs and distended bellies; the almost dead and the dead. But even more horrifying was the stench, the foul and constant odor of soldiers mangled by war.

Compared to the world wars that followed it, the Franco-Prussian War seems insignificant now, of interest only to archivists of nineteenth-century maps showing long-obsolete borders. Yet in fact it was a seminal conflict. Though it lasted less than a year, it was the prototype for the wars of the twentieth century in terms of the issues behind the conflict (the taut borders of Europe and the influence of overseas dominions and resources), the scale of its battles (these could involve hundreds of thousands of troops at once), and the conditions faced by soldiers on the front lines (for the first time, rifles and cannons were accurate and massively deadly). And like few wars before but all wars since, it served as a laboratory for medicine, creating a rich opportunity for physician-scientists to study the grotesque impact of new weaponry on the human body and the effectiveness, or lack thereof, of efforts to treat those injured so horribly.

In their way, the weapons deployed for this conflict were beautifully designed specimens of breakthrough technology. The Germans deployed the newly patented Krupp cannon, which could be loaded from the breech rather than the front. The Krupp made it possible to fire six-pound shells far more quickly than France's muzzle-loading cannon, meaning more missiles exploding in the air, raining a heavier barrage of zinc shrapnel down upon French troops. (The Germans also made history by deploying the first antiaircraft guns, firing at French balloons.) For their part, the French army debuted the *mitrailleuse*, an early mounted machine gun that could fire a hundred rounds per minute—a barrage the German troops called the "battle squirt." As an 1873 report on the war described it, "The growling of this 'wild beast of battle' resembles nothing so much as the running of an anchor cable through a ship's cathead, or the closing of heavy iron shutters."

But though the *mitrailleuse* made a terrifying noise, it inflicted fairly few of the casualties showing up at Koch's hospital. The real agent of destruction was the French rifle, the chassepot, a rapid-fire, high-velocity rifle that could be accurate from a stunning 1,200 meters away (nearly three-quarters of a mile). It was, as one German officer described it, "a gorgeously worked murder weapon." (The Germans were equipped with their patented needle gun, an older, less impressive piece of technology that could fire from only 700 meters, creating what was called the chassepot gap, where French troops could hit the Germans, but not vice versa.)

Unlike in previous wars, where the rifles created the soundtrack but the bayonet did most of the damage, in this war there were remarkably few wounds from knifepoint. Rather, the wounded soldiers that Koch and his colleagues tended to bore the unique scars of long-range rifle shots: diffuse, open wounds with splintered bone fragments and bits of clothing mixed in with the damaged flesh. Most of the soldiers who came in to the hospital bore limb wounds, as those with wounds to the abdomen usually died on the battlefield. Amputation was the routine treatment, and a miserable death from gangrene the routine result.

Ether, thankfully, was now available to surgeons, having been invented twenty-five years before, but still, the typical procedure was brutal and fast. The surgeon would fix on the wound, pick the opportune place to separate the limb, and then hack through it with a saw. An amputation was over in less than a minute; a skilled hand could finish in twenty-five seconds. If the soldier was lucky, the surgeon took care to leave enough skin intact to fix a flap over the stump.

Charles Alexander Gordon, an English doctor observing hospital conditions during the war, described a German facility this way:

> It was not an unfrequent sight to see the blood and discharges from wounds soaking into the bedding, where they speedily underwent decomposition, and thus became sources of various evils, producing at the same time a most offensive and sickening odour.
>
> Patients were left for many hours in the clothes in which they had been wounded, and such was the pressure of the times, that clothing, after being taken off patients, has been left lying in the wards for 36 and even 48 hours afterwards, giving out offensiveness.

Still, despite such appalling conditions, the Germans were in far better shape than the French. For one thing, Germany had made better preparations at the outset. They recruited 5,548 physicians for the war effort, 3,000 nurses, and nearly 500 apothecaries. The French, on the other hand, had barely 1,000 available surgeons when the war began, and fewer nurses and other staff in turn. Germany, too, had taken some essential preventive measures, mandating smallpox vaccines for all new troops. The French had no such requirement, with devastating consequences. While fewer than 300 German soldiers died of smallpox, the inevitable outbreak on the French side eventually claimed the lives of 25,000 troops. (In a demonstration of the ancillary costs of war, the epidemic subsequently spread to civilian populations on both sides of the new border in France and Germany. This time Germany paid the higher price, with 177,000 civilian fatalities to France's 90,000.)

The Prussian advantage went beyond preparations. In treatment and recovery, too, German troops fared better—chiefly because their commanders had subscribed to the methods of the Scottish surgeon Joseph Lister, who a few years earlier had developed the principle of "antiseptic surgery" against the threat of germs. In the civilian world, the germ theory—the idea that some disease was caused by microscopic agents, or germs, that would release toxins and attack the body—was a radical notion. It contradicted the conventional wisdom that disease was a product of bad air, or miasma. But on the battlefield, such disputes were academic. Lister had demonstrated that his approach saved lives, so the Germans, keenly aware that disease had historically always been more deadly to military forces than actual battle, made Lister's antiseptic procedure compulsory at all medical facilities.

By today's standards, Lister's treatment was coarse, even brutal. It looked nothing like today's sterile surgical environment, with its stainless-steel basins and bright lights, everyone swathed head to toe in pristine blue scrubs. Surgeons weren't even required to wash their equipment or hands. Rather, Lister's antisepsis took for granted that a doctor's hands would be filthy with the last patient's blood and guts and that instruments would be poorly cleaned. His new technique called for a doctor to douse a wound with a dilution of carbolic acid, otherwise known as phenol, an extract of coal tar. In German facilities, this took the form of what was called Lister's cerate: one part crystallized carbolic acid, six parts linseed oil, nine parts chalk. Bandages, too, would be soaked in the stuff before wounds were dressed. It was a caustic, painful bath. (Today phenol is used in paint stripper, among other things.) Many surgeons disliked Lister's cerate because its use made procedures take longer; an amputation was harder to dispatch in thirty seconds when there was so much dousing and swabbing to be done. But the results were real and demonstrable. Antisepsis did the job, killing many of the bacteria in and around the wound. As Dr. Gordon observed, "this preparation, spread upon tinfoil . . . proved to be both convenient and effective." Though the German hospitals were far from clean, the measures the Germans did take would prove revolutionary. In fact, for the first time in any war, the Germans would be the first to lose more men directly to battle wounds than to subsequent infection.

The French, meanwhile, followed the principles of François Broussais, a renowned French physician from earlier in the century. Alas, Broussais's work was woefully out of date—he was a firm believer in bleeding by leeches—and had disastrous consequences for the French side. Whereas Lister's cerate eliminated bacteria, Broussais's technique was to apply salves to open wounds in the hope of soothing inflammation. In the French hospitals, open jars of greasy ointment lined the shelves behind an operating table, ready for the surgeon to scoop out a dollop with his unwashed hands, wiping the stuff into the patient's wound. With the next patient, he'd go back to the same tub with the same dirty hand. One couldn't have designed a better procedure for disseminating infectious disease, and the results bore this out: of 13,173 amputations performed in French military hospitals, 10,006 ended in death, a fatality rate of nearly 70 percent. (One wonders if the survival rate would have been better if they'd just left the mangled limbs attached.)

Hospital disease was the catch-all term for any infection that befell patients outside battle, and it was common in both German and French facilities. Some cases were classified as pyemia (a severe fever known today as sepsis, where the blood is poisoned by *Staphylococcus* infection), others were gangrene (where an infection starts to kill large amounts of tissue), and still others were typhoid or typhus (a fever that appeared symptomatically, like typhoid, though it was spread by lice harboring *Rickettsia* bacterium). Whatever the classification, when a merely wounded soldier developed a hospital disease, he was considered effectively lost. In German field hospitals such as Koch's, these patients were moved into their own wards, since the illness did seem to spread from the sick to the not-yet-sick. Whether this quarantine was motivated by a belief in germs or simply in bad air, it was the reality of the battlefield. As Dr. Gordon observed, "In this war, as in all others, it has been shown that, wherever large accumulations of wounded took place, there pyaemia, in one form or other, appeared, and proved as fatal as it had ever done."

Though the infections meant misery and near-certain death for soldiers, they offered a morbid opportunity for enterprising physicians, none more than Edwin Klebs, a Prussian physician a decade older than Koch. Klebs was stationed in Karlsruhe, a German border city near Strasbourg, and, like Koch, attended to cases in the town's railroad depot, which had been converted to a hospital. In addition to the requisite surgeries and amputations, Klebs also performed autopsies on fallen soldiers.

One afternoon, out of curiosity, he slipped some tissue from a fatal gunshot wound under a microscope. What he saw through the lens amazed him. "I found rod-shaped bodies, so-called bacteria," Klebs wrote in a subsequent report, noting that these organisms increased in number when present with pus and fever. Significantly, he observed that they weren't all identical, but rather comprised some smaller sporelike shapes in clumps, some rods, and others somewhere in between. So far, Klebs's observation was simply an association—he'd noticed that these bodies appeared along with infection; others before him had made similar observations. But then Klebs took a bold leap from association to causation, proposing an actual relationship between the bacteria and the infection: He asserted that the one *created* the other. "These parasitical organisms are the cause of severe manifestations," he declared. His methodology here was sound if not airtight: First he noted that the bacteria appeared in every instance of open, inflamed wounds. Second, he also tried to reproduce the bacteria in cultures. This was only somewhat successful, since his samples were generally contaminated.

Klebs was on the right path: The bacteria were the cause of the pus, the fever, and the infection at root. But his proposal was not convincing. He lacked a definitive chain of evidence that might convince his colleagues and overturn the orthodoxy that inflammation was caused by internal mechanisms of the cells, a theory advanced, most notably, by Rudolf Virchow, the leading pathologist of Europe (and former mentor to Klebs). Klebs might have made the jump from association to causation, but his profession would not follow—at least not yet. As a surgeon reviewing Klebs's report remarked, "Does disease follow bacteria, or do bacteria follow disease? We still don't know the answer."

AMONG THE PRUSSIAN MEDICAL STAFF, KLEBS WAS AN EXCEPTION, not only because he had the wherewithal to pull out his microscope, but also because, in his station hospital, with its stone walls, granite floors, and solid roof, he had the relative luxury to do so. Back in the field hospitals, physicians such as Koch were sunk too deep in the slop of war to think about science. But Koch wasn't intimidated by the horrors he witnessed. In his few months, he enthusiastically wrote to his father, he had learned more than in all his prior surgical training. Finally his life had a purpose, a focus, an outcome. "I will never regret the decision to participate in this war. Apart from the scientific experiences that I had gained—worth more than 6 months in a clinic—I have gained much experience in life. This will serve me well in coming years."

Still, by mid-January, Koch had grown concerned that his practice in Rackwitz was in jeopardy, and he made an official request to be sent back. It was quickly granted. A few months later, the entire Franco-Prussian War was over, not a year after it had begun. That was long enough, still, to claim some 170,000 lives: 30,000 German and 140,000 French.

Robert Koch returned to Emma and daughter, Gertrud, in Rackwitz and resumed his medical practice. It was as if the war had never happened. At twenty-seven, he again began to suspect that his life was settling into stasis. Then he received an invitation from the Baron von Unruhe-Bomst—whom he had treated for that gunshot wound a couple of years before—to take up a government position as the local health officer in Wöllstein, a town to the north. By April 1872, Koch and family were on the move again.

Wöllstein, an agricultural town of three thousand in eastern Germany tucked between two lakes, had a history dating to 1458. (Today the town sits in western Poland and is known as Wolsztyn.) For centuries it had been a center for sheep farming and wool production. In the 1870s, wool was the world's leading textile, and Germany the largest producer, with Wöllstein, which means "wool stones," as a hub.

Koch settled his family into 12 Strasse am weissen Berge ("Road to the White Mountain"), a large Gothic building almost dead center in the town that had previously functioned as a hospital for the poor. Upstairs were the living quarters: four rooms and a kitchen, with a large bay window over the street. Koch's examination room was downstairs. Out back was a garden, filled with trees and flowers, where his daughter could run around.

Koch thrived in Wöllstein. His neighbors trusted him and kept him busy with smallpox vaccinations, injuries and illnesses, and aches and pains. The days were long but full. Emma was happier, too, and proved to be a diligent doctor's wife, handling patients and minding the family budget. After a few months, she proudly told her husband that she'd saved enough to buy something for the practice. She suggested either a carriage, which would make his visits to patients much easier, scattered as they were throughout the countryside, or a new microscope. He chose the scope.

THE MICROSCOPE WAS FIRST DEVELOPED IN THE SEVENTEENTH CENTURY by fixing a single lens onto a stand, with an assist from a nearby candle. The instrument's first great demonstration was Robert Hooke's *Micrographia*. Published in 1665 by the Royal Society in London, Hooke's book is said to be the first scientific bestseller. The diarist Samuel Pepys, who bought a copy he saw in the window of his local bookshop, wrote that he stayed up until two in the morning reading it, calling it "the most ingenious book I read in my life." Hooke was the first to use the word *cells* to describe the pores in wood; he thought they looked like a monk's room, or cell. The thirty-eight plates in his book, many of them massive drawings that the reader had to unfold to see in full, showed meticulous hand drawings of fleas, gnats, and lice in exquisite detail. The precision is remarkable even now, as is Hooke's written description:

> By the means of Telescopes, there is nothing so far distant but may be represented to our view; and by the help of Microscopes, there is nothing so small, as to escape our inquiry; hence there is a new visible World discovered to the understanding. By this means the Heavens are open'd, and a vast number of new Stars, and new Motions, and new Productions appear in them, to which all the ancient Astronomers were utterly Strangers. By this the Earth it self, which lyes so

neer us, under our feet, shews quite a new thing to us, and in
every little particle of its matter, we now behold almost as
great a variety of creatures as we were able before to reckon
up on the whole Universe it self.

Hooke was soon on to experiments with telescopes and gravity
(his research preceded Newton's by a decade, the grounds of a long-
standing grudge between the two men). But his microscopic discoveries were soon elaborated by Antonie van Leeuwenhoek, a Dutchman
who was too much a tinkerer to be satisfied with pondering insect
anatomy. Van Leeuwenhoek improved upon Hooke's microscope by
adding a small glass bead as a lens, thus amplifying the tool's resolution. His lens-grinding technique could achieve a magnifying
power of 266 times, allowing him to discern features just .00135 mil-
limeters apart. Soon, van Leeuwenhoek was peering beyond the anatomical to the cellular, sketching out the parts of blood, human
spermatozoa, and various animalcules.

It would be more than a century and a half before microscopes
were significantly improved. In the 1820s, Joseph Jackson Lister, the
father of the antiseptic surgeon, began experimenting with how a
second lens could bend an image back upon itself and increase the
microscope's power accordingly. Twenty years later the German lens
makers Carl Zeiss perfected the industrial manufacture of the tool,
allowing economies of scale to kick in. Leeuwenhoek had made it
powerful, Lister made it reliable, and Carl Zeiss made it affordable:
Those three components allowed the technology to flourish.

The microscope was one of several technological instruments to
reach medicine in the nineteenth century. The stethoscope, which allowed physicians to hear inside the chest, was the first; a version was
invented in 1816. It was followed, in 1851, by the ophthalmoscope,
which made it possible for the first time to see inside the human eye,
creating the modern specialty of ophthalmology. Other scopes, all invented around the same time, had a similar impact: the otoscope for

the ears; the endoscope for the gut. Each of these scopes made it possible for the physician to see inside the patient, to push past the limitations of the patient's physiology and the physician's senses. (They were all upstaged by the discovery of X-rays in 1895, by Wilhelm Roentgen, which radically altered the physician's perception of the patient.) When the stethoscope was perfected into its now-iconic form and function in the 1850s, for instance, it made it possible for a physician to hear a patient's lungs and heart, connecting various sounds inside with various symptoms on the outside. It became especially indispensable as a tool for the diagnosis and assessment of tuberculosis.

All these scopes would be described today as disruptive technologies: They rattled the status quo of nineteenth-century clinical care, in particular the physician. Most were suspicious of the new tools, which seemed to encroach on their authority. This distrust was nicely captured by Dr. Oliver Wendell Holmes, in his day the most respected physician in the United States, and a respected poet. In a bit of verse called "The Stethoscope Song," published in 1848, Dr. Holmes lampooned a wet-behind-the-ears doctor enthralled by his fancy new stethoscope, which leads him to mistake a buzzing fly for a patient's heartbeat.

In truth, the arrival of the scopes marked a significant shift toward the scientific practice of medicine and away from the inherited art of medicine. "Learn to see microscopically," the German pathologist Rudolf Virchow often said, imploring his students at the University of Berlin to master the craft of close observation and analysis. Virchow, the most celebrated physician of the day, was a fierce advocate for the widespread adoption of microscopy in medicine. It was a lesson that Robert Koch would take to heart, to the eventual chagrin even of the great Virchow.

BY 1873, KOCH'S PRACTICE WAS FLOURISHING. HE TREATED RINGWORM and dysentery, whooping cough and colic, and aches and infections and attended births and deaths. During spare hours, he would go down to the lakes and bottle up some water samples. Back home, he'd examine them under his microscope, noting the microorganisms he observed. And on idle afternoons, he and his friend the baron would pack up shovels and trowels and visit nearby prehistoric settlements, digging into ancient Teutonic graves.

On one such excursion, Koch discovered a trove of ancient relics. Knowing that Rudolf Virchow shared his interest in archaeology, Koch sent a note inviting him to Wöllstein to see the find. They spent a pleasant morning inspecting the dig, and Virchow arranged for some of the artifacts to be displayed in Berlin.

In Berlin, Virchow ran the new Institute of Pathology at the Charité, the illustrious medical center. There, he devised his cell theory of disease, which argued that all cells come from preexisting cells, refuting the false notion of spontaneous generation of disease. Unfortunately, Virchow proposed a new fallacy: that the body generated its own disease. "Disease is nothing but life under altered conditions," he stated. He believed that epidemic disease was inextricably social, and advocated hygienic measures decades before they became commonplace.

The German word for science is *Wissenschaft*, which literally means creating systematic knowledge; it requires an application of a method, a process. In the nineteenth century, *Wissenschaft* became the official ideology of German universities, an institutional demand upon every student and professor that they pursue their research with rigor, thoroughness, and care. Virchow especially thrilled to this larger task. "Die Medicin ist eine sociale Wissenschaft," he wrote, meaning that medicine had the potential for profound social impact. "We shall soon perceive that observation and experiments only have a permanent value," he wrote in 1847. "Then, not as the outgrowth of personal enthusiasm, but as the result of the labors of many close investigators, pathological physiology will find its sphere. It will prove the fortress of scientific medicine, the outworks of which are pathological anatomy and clinical research."

Virchow was his own finest example: He published thousands of scientific papers during his fifty-year career, covering everything from a taxonomy of parasites to a catalog of the shapes of the heads of German schoolboys, from leprosy in Norway to swamp diseases in ancient Troy. It's hard to overstate the shadow Virchow cast over German medicine; he appeared to have taken it, single-handedly, and thrust it into modernity. In the 1870s, three decades after his first calls for scientific medicine, Virchow wrote that "it is no longer necessary today to write that scientific medicine is also the best foundation for medical practice," though he evidently felt compelled to write it nonetheless. "Even the external character of medical practice has changed in the last thirty years. Scientific methods have been everywhere introduced into practice."

As a student, Koch arrived at Göttingen just as Virchow's call to arms was beginning to seem self-evident. With the diligent example of teachers such as Henle, Koch would have been indoctrinated with this sense of history and opportunity. But where Virchow looked in his scope and could see only cells of human origin, Henle saw microbes.

Like the proverbial blind men touching the elephant, both Virchow and Henle were partly right and partly wrong. Virchow's dogmatism for cell theory helped push medicine toward science and away from humoral theory; in his way he was as much a radical as Koch would become. For his part, Henle was correct to put faith in microscopy (in what could be seen) and to evangelize against miasma and for germs. He was undoubtedly on the right path when he suggested that "before microscopic forms can be regarded as the cause of contagion in men, they must be constantly found in the contagious material; they must be isolated from it and their strength tested." The statement would become the blueprint for Koch's career.

WÖLLSTEIN IS JUST 230 KILOMETERS, OR 140 MILES, FROM BERLIN. But in the 1870s, 230 kilometers might as well have been 230,000. If Koch yearned for better prospects, there seemed no way to leave Wöllstein. He had a solid practice, and his patients admired him. Given his meager background, he had indeed arrived. Except that he had arrived in Wöllstein, such as it was.

So rather than look to Berlin, Koch looked to Wöllstein. In 1873, just as he began to grow bored of looking at pond water under his scope, a new opportunity to test his science emerged. Sheep in the area had begun to die. Then a few local farmers and sheep shearers began to get sick as well. This happened from time to time in such a place, an outbreak of a malady known as woolsorter's disease. It was also called anthrax.

Historically, anthrax was a common, and devastating, part of agriculture. Farmers called it the "black bane" and could only watch as the disease ran its course from symptoms to death in a matter of hours. An infected animal would slow down, drift back from the herd, and soon fall to the ground. Blood would stream from the mouth and nose. And just like that, the animal would be dead. Inside the swollen cadaver, the organs would be awash in a dark fluid, and the spleen, in particular, would be distended.

In humans, anthrax on the skin was unmistakable: Boils with a dark, almost black, center of necrotic flesh would break out on the hands and arms, and red streaks would spread up and down the affected limb. It is an ugly, disfiguring infection, and before the discovery of antibiotics, it would prove fatal in about 15 percent of cases.

Anthrax is an ancient disease; biblical scholars have suggested that it was the fifth plague on Egypt. "Behold, the hand of the Lord is upon thy cattle which is in the field, upon the horses, upon the asses, upon the camels, upon the oxen, and upon the sheep," the King James Bible describes. "There shall be a very grievous murrain."

For farmers in any era, the disease spelled disaster. But in the late nineteenth century, when the cattle, wool, and leather industries had become integral components of a booming European economy, the disease was especially unwelcome. In 1870 in Russia, where the disease was known as the "Siberian pest," an outbreak in Novograd killed 56,000 cattle and 528 people. Anthrax was endemic in Italy; in the ten years from 1880 to 1890 there were more than 24,000 reported human cases, with nearly 6,000 fatalities.

The cause was a great mystery. A French veterinarian suggested that anthrax in sheep was brought about by an excess of blood circulating in the vessels, due to too much feeding. Others believed the disease was in fact poisoning by a toxic plant, though which plant could never be determined. Others simply thought that the fields themselves were cursed.

When the Wöllstein outbreak took hold in late 1873 and began spreading to humans as well as sheep, Koch probably used the available folk remedies: poultices of cow manure or tree bark, leaves, and even roasted onion. He may have treated some wounds with surgery, excising the diseased flesh or cauterizing it with a hot iron or acid. From time to time, though, he would take the blood from a recently stricken animal and put it under his microscope. On April 12, 1874, he described what he saw in his notebook. There were spores, some of which grew into chains of rods—these must be bacteria, he wrote, using the term that the German zoologist Christian Gottfried Ehrenberg had coined in 1838 to describe tiny rod-shaped organisms. "The bacteria swell up, become shinier, thicker, and much longer," he observed.

Koch wasn't the first scientist to look at the strange, dark blood of a dead animal through a microscope and observe these bacteria. Anthrax, as it happens, is a particularly large bacterium, easy to see under a scope. In 1850 the French physicians Casamir Davaine and Pierre Rayer observed "little, threadlike motionless bodies" in the blood of sheep that had died of anthrax. Though he couldn't determine whether these bodies were living or dead, Davaine went on to show that the blood of one animal with the disease could infect another, and he conjectured that these "bacteridia" were the cause of the disease. The German physician Aloys Pollender recorded a similar observation in 1855 and in his report likewise speculated about bacteria's link to disease. "Whether they are the infectious material itself or simply the bearers of it, or, perhaps, have no connection with it at all?"

This, of course, was the essential question. Did these microbes cause disease or were they caused by it? Or were they mere bystanders? It's the question that made Klebs's battlefield research so suggestive but ultimately unconvincing. As one surgeon said in reaction to Klebs's work, "My heart says 'yes' to bacteria, but my reason says 'wait, wait.'" It was a true mystery of cause and effect, and dozens of scientists, with better resources and training than Koch, had failed to solve it. Why should Koch, sitting in his kitchen in Wöllstein, be any different?

That summer, the anthrax outbreak seemed to wane. As the months passed, Koch fell back into his routine practice—but his passion for the microscopic world only grew. Emma had saved enough money to buy another, better microscope, which Koch would use long into the night, examining blood from the animals out back, even bits of tissue from his patients.

A year went by, and Koch went back to his practice. Then, a few days before Christmas 1875, a local police officer came across a dead animal near town. The beast's blood was dark and thick, a sure sign of anthrax. Fearing another outbreak, the officer took the dead animal to Dr. Koch, who extracted some blood and placed it under his microscope. Sure enough, it was teeming with the bacteria he had noted eighteen months before. He found himself in just the same place, facing just the same question: Were these bacteria the cause of disease or the result? Once again, Koch considered the question, mulling it over.

Then he began an experiment.

CHAPTER 2

1875 · The Germ Theory

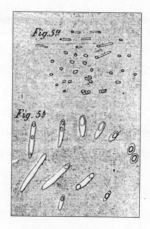

Sketch by Robert Koch of Bacillus anthracis, *from his 1876 paper*

Koch's first experiment, on the evening of December 23, 1875, was remarkably simple: He went outside to his garden, pulled a healthy rabbit out of its cage, and brought it back to his makeshift laboratory downstairs. He drew a sample of the animal's blood and examined it under his microscope, making sure it was clear of the bacteria he'd seen earlier in dead animals. Then he took some blood from the corpse the police officer had brought over and injected it into the ear of the rabbit.

Koch spent the following day tending to a full office of patients, and that evening, when he looked in the cage, the rabbit was dead. He removed its ear, cut off some tissue, and examined it under the microscope. The bacteria were there, "in moderate numbers," Koch observed in his notebook.

The next day was Christmas. Wöllstein was quiet as families celebrated the holiday at home. On Strasse am weissen Berge, Emma
was preparing a holiday dinner upstairs, with Gertrud nearby. Downstairs, Koch was oblivious to the occasion. With no patients to attend
to, he'd spent all day on his research. He removed some other tissue
from the dead rabbit and found that it had even more bacteria than
the day before; clearly these germs were reproducing. It wasn't quite
cause and effect, but the creatures were thriving. In his notebook, he
planned a series of experiments that he hoped would link the bacteria
to the disease.

The following day, the patients returned. But Koch's evenings
were spent in the quiet laboratory. He injected one healthy mouse
with blood from one that had been sick. When the new one died, he
injected its blood into another mouse, and so on and so on, until
twenty mice had passed along both the bacteria and the disease. "In
all the animals the results were the same," he wrote in his notebook,
keeping assiduous track of every step. "The spleen was markedly
swollen in appearance and contained a large number of transparent
rods which were very similar in appearance."

Koch knew it wasn't enough just to inject animals with infected
blood. Davaine had followed that path in his experiments a few years
before and had still failed to prove his case. Koch would have to go
further. He would have to conduct a series of experiments that, with
each step, established a chain of evidence that irrefutably connected
the bacterium with the disease.

This began, Koch realized, with Henle's directive: to create a
culture of the bacteria. Only by growing the microbes in something
other than a living animal could he be certain his experiment was not
polluted by something undetectable in the animal. The tricky part
here was finding a medium for the growth. Many before had tried to
nudge the anthrax bacteria to grow outside an animal, but they had
failed.

Koch's solution was ingenious: the hanging drop. First, he took a cattle eye he'd procured from the local slaughterhouse, and drained the fluid, known as aqueous humor. In this fluid he placed a sample of spleen from a mouse that had died of anthrax. Then he placed a drop of the fluid on a thin slide, and fit this slide over a thicker slide into which he'd carved a small concave well. He lined the slides with petroleum jelly and pressed them together, forming a sealed environment for the drop of fluid, which hung in the chamber. He put the slides under his microscope and had a look.

For an hour, then two, nothing happened. The spleen tissue seemed to sit, inert, in the cattle-eye humor. Then, suddenly, the sticks of bacteria began to divide and grow. After a few hours, the whole drop was filled with microbes. They were clearly alive, and they were clearly growing in this novel medium. The chain of evidence was falling into place, and Koch's notebooks grew thick with drawings of *Bacillus anthracis*, the whorls of filaments covering the pages.

As Koch's experiments went on, his backyard menagerie began to thin out; his daughter, Gertrud, grew concerned that she was losing all her pets. He needed a new pool of animals to experiment upon. Koch and Emma set live mousetraps in the horse barn behind their house. They caught a bounty and stuffed them into tall glass jars with some holes poked in the lid for air. When he needed an animal, he'd pull one out, tail first, using an old bullet extractor he'd saved from the war. After the mouse had died, ostensibly from the microbes, Koch would dissect it, searching for the bacteria—and then dispose of the cadaver by burning it in the oven. Later, he found a more dependable source of animals, after a friend sent Gertrud some white mice as pets. The animals began reproducing rapidly, and Koch began using the extra supply in his lab. These became one of his most iconic contributions to science: the white lab mouse.

By this point, Koch needed some dedicated space for his experiments. He took a heavy brown curtain and hung it across the ceiling of his examination room, dividing it in two: one side was for patients, and the other served as his laboratory. As soon as he was done seeing patients, he would cross behind the curtain and turn to his experiments, staying up long into the night. Working without electricity, he struggled to maintain the right temperature to grow his cultures. Soon he devised a layered element of sand, paper, and glass that he could place over a low flame. The technique maintained the culture at a steady ninety degrees Fahrenheit—an ideal climate for home-brewed anthrax. In this way, his one experiment contained a multitude of smaller experiments, a pyramid of challenges Koch had to solve one by one in order to work toward the larger question of causality.

He began to buy more equipment: a new, more powerful microscope; a spectroscope; and a microtome (an instrument for cutting small tissue samples). He began to skirt appointments and beg off house calls in town in order to do one more experiment, to check one more mouse spleen under the microscope. Emma found herself running interference for her distracted husband. "It was my job to find out first how sick a patient really was," she explained to her father, "and to send away those who didn't really need medical attention. In that way, Robert could often remain for hours at his work."

Koch's research began suggesting a larger discovery than just causality between a microbe and a disease. He was, in fact, composing a portrait of the entire life cycle of the organism, a chronicle of its various stages, and the deadliness of the bacteria at each stage—because the bacteria, he had observed, weren't just static long rods. They would swell and grow, forming long filaments. Those filaments shot off round spores that had materially different qualities from the rods. For instance, when a sample of rods was dried under heat, they would be rendered inert; injected into an animal, they would not produce disease. But the spores were hardier structures. Even after being heated and dried out, when introduced into the aqueous humor, they would awaken and generate new rods and new spheres.

This, Koch began to realize, was the true secret of the bacteria's deadly power. In spore form, anthrax can remain dormant for years, waiting for a suitable host—a grazing sheep, say—to come ͟. was how anthrax could emerge, as if from the sky—becau͟ simply stayed well hidden in the ground.

By April he was convinced that he had sufficient eviden͟. He had isolated the bacteria—which he would call *Bacillus anthracis*—in a dead animal, reproduced it in a culture, inoculated it into a healthy animal, and then, after that animal quickly died, found the bacteria in the blood, in plentitude. He had isolated the dormant spores and shown how they could be revived in culture. It was a clear demonstration of causation, one that pinpointed the very mechanism of the disease, and one that had never been demonstrated so thoroughly, exhaustively, or repeatedly. As he summarized in his notes, "In view of this fact, all doubts as to whether the Bacillus anthracis is really the cause and contagium of anthrax just fall silent." He had succeeded, he said, "for the first time to shed light on the etiology of one of these strange diseases."

But if Koch had proven this to himself, he now faced an even more daunting task: How could he, a thirty-two-year-old country doctor, possibly convince the world? How could he even begin to communicate what he had discovered?

KOCH'S RESOURCES MIGHT HAVE BEEN MEAGER, HIS TECHNIQUE improvisational, but the question he'd answered stood as one of humanity's most enduring mysteries: What causes disease? What are the mechanisms behind the ills that afflict us?

For centuries the question had a straightforward, if increasingly unsatisfying answer. The ancient Greek physician Hippocrates proposed that the four humors (phlegm, black bile, yellow bile, and blood) governed all human health; disease was caused by an imbalance among these humors. In AD 150 the theory was endorsed and elaborated upon by Galen, and well into the nineteenth century, humoral medicine remained the status quo. It wasn't until Virchow, with his revolutionary theory of cellular pathology, that humors would be pushed aside. But even he couldn't fathom such a thing as germs.

Here and there, though, an outspoken contrarian had peered through his microscope and seen a new way to explain disease. In the 1840s the Hungarian physician Ignaz Semmelweis was practicing in the General Hospital in Vienna. At the time, death in childbirth was a real worry, with about 5 percent of expectant mothers dying while giving birth, many from puerperal fever, known as "childbirth fever," following delivery. The General Hospital had two maternity wards, divided by class: in the first, elite patients received care from physicians and medical students; in the second ward, lower classes were attended to by midwives. Semmelweis monitored the two clinics and found that, to his surprise, the death rate was far higher in the first ward than in the second. Fully 13 percent of women attended to by medical staff died, while just 2 percent of women with midwives did.

Faced with these numbers, Semmelweis came to a horrific realization: The medical students were working on cadavers in the hospital morgue barehanded and then attending to the expectant mothers directly afterward, without washing their hands between. As they moved from corpse to mother, they carried the germs (which would later be identified as *Staphylococcus* and *Streptococcus*) with them.

Semmelweis soon demonstrated a solution: He required that medical students wash their hands in a lime-chlorine solution after their autopsies. The process dramatically reduced fatalities in the first ward, putting them on par with those in the midwife ward. But that was as far as Semmelweis's discovery went. In 1849 he was deemed too controversial and refused a reappointment at the hospital. He would spend the next years railing against medical standards and evangelizing against germs, but the medical establishment was unconvinced. Semmelweis would die in an insane asylum in 1865, tormented by the agony of having his work thrown on the rubbish heap. His tragedy, as the writer Céline would later write, was that "his discovery was too great for the strength of his genius."

But germs kept revealing themselves and kept tempt⸱
join the argument for the contagiousness of disease. In
glishman John Grove published a treatise whose very title m⸱
argument: *Epidemics Examined and Explained: Or, Living Germ⸱
Proved by Analogy to Be a Source of Disease*—the "by Analogy" being
Grove's admission that, though he had the argument, he lacked the
evidence. A few years later, an outbreak of cholera in London drew
John Snow to investigate; he famously demonstrated that contaminated drinking water, rather than miasma, was the conduit for the
disease. Today, Snow is celebrated for his symbolic victory in having
the handle removed from the culprit pump, and as the father of epidemiology. But in fact, his larger efforts to improve sanitation in London
were thwarted.

Most prominently of all, there was Louis Pasteur, who in the
1850s and '60s offered remarkable evidence that microbes caused fermentation and spoilage. The work launched Pasteur on a crusade
against spontaneous generation and led him to claim boldly in 1864
that "life is a germ, and a germ is life." The germ theory finally had its
great champion. But Pasteur's evidence, alas, stemmed almost entirely
from food and industry, not human disease. The connection between
the two was neither explicit nor obvious, which made Pasteur's claims,
once again, conjecture. It wasn't until Joseph Lister built on Pasteur's
work with his techniques for antiseptic surgery in the 1860s that the
worlds began to align. Lister's work convinced some surgeons to adopt
sterilization methods, though theirs was largely a practical capitulation,
not a philosophical one. Others remained recalcitrant. "Where are
these little beasts?" scoffed John Hughes Bennett, a medical professor
at Edinburgh. "Show them to us, and we shall believe in them. Has
anyone seen them yet?"

By the 1870s, many scientists, including Klebs and Henle, were
hard at work conducting research that might prove the germ theory
and preaching the new gospel at every opportunity. In 1877, Klebs was
confident enough to maintain, in a talk entitled "On the Revolution in

Medical Opinions in the Last Three Decades," that most diseases considered routine were likely to be contagious—that is, caused by germs. If the germs "are found exclusively in the given disease process," he explained, then "it can be decisive to convey the disease by means of organisms that have been isolated and cultivated outside the body." Even tuberculosis, he maintained, was likely caused by germs.

But Klebs's laboratory efforts, time and again, fell short of a more thorough proof, leaving his exhortations thrilling but unconvincing rhetoric. Lacking certain evidence, the germ theory would remain a radical idea, outside the mainstream of medicine. Then as now, the principle of Occam's razor prevailed: The simplest explanation wins out, and the notion of germs causing disease was too fantastic, too contrary to everything otherwise understood, to displace the prevailing understanding of disease.

From today's vantage point, it's possible to see why the first wave of germ theorists failed to convince their peers of the certainty of their ideas. In each of these cases, the argument for germs was based on association and proximity. Each proposed a theory, offered some evidence, and made his argument. But there were too many holes and gaps, too much rhetorical hand waving. They were snagged on the shoals of the hypothetical, the if-it-were-possibles that had stymied Henle. Even Pasteur, who had worked for years to debunk the theory of spontaneous generation, seemed unable to marshal the chain of evidence that would uproot orthodoxy and convince the establishment that germs offered a simpler, more likely explanation.

Lacking that clear chain toward causation, rather than mere association, it was too easy for the scientific status quo, not to mention the public at large, to reject the germ theory outright. Surely the idea of some secret world of tiny creatures, bent on killing us, was more outlandish than the evidence that lay before us: that the air itself was bad, and that as vapors spread, so did disease. That idea, known as miasma, sounded like common sense. As the scientific journal *La Presse* editorialized to Pasteur in 1860, "I am afraid that the experiments you quote,

M. Pasteur, will turn against you. The world into which you wish to take us is really too fantastic."

In his book *The Structure of Scientific Revolutions*, written in 1962, Thomas Kuhn proposed a new way to look at science: not as the inevitable, persistent discovery of truth, but rather as "the piecemeal process by which . . . items are added, singly and in combination, to the ever growing stockpile that constitutes scientific technique and knowledge." That piecemeal process typically happens slowly, in what Kuhn calls "normal science." But it can also happen with a start, in an explosion of new research and new knowledge that upsets the stockpile (the status quo) with a new paradigm for understanding the world. New science, Kuhn argued, needs to be powerful enough not just to prove its point, but also to overwhelm the traditions that already explain the world.

Kuhn's essay was revolutionary in its own right for reframing the perception of how science happens. He suggested that this was not a smooth, regular process toward progress; it was traumatic and destructive and could be downright threatening. Though Kuhn, a physicist by training, was concerned mostly about revolutions in astronomy and physics—Newton's discoveries, Einstein's theory of relativity, and such—his framework applies very well to the germ theory and to Koch's and Pasteur's efforts to prove a valid, if revolutionary, framework for understanding disease.

Kuhn's point was that any revolution inevitably comes down to an overthrow, and that can be an especially difficult task when the opposition is other scientists. As Bernard Barber put it just a year before Kuhn, in a 1961 *Science* essay entitled "Resistance by Scientists to Scientific Discovery," "as men in society, scientists are sometimes the agents, sometimes the objects, of resistance to their own discoveries." For the would-be revolutionary, this obstinacy can be infuriating, and even, as Semmelweis showed, maddening.

As one of those early germ theory revolutionaries, Lister bore the scars from his fights with the conventional wisdom. In an address to graduating medical students in 1877, he urged them to beware the easy temptation to reject an unfamiliar idea.

> In investigating nature you will do well to bear ever in mind that in every question there is the truth, whatever our notions may be. This seems perhaps a very simple consideration, yet it is strange how often it seems to be disregarded. I remember at an early period of my own life showing to a man of high reputation as a teacher some matters which I happened to have observed. And I was very much struck, and grieved, to find that while all the facts lay equally clear before him, those only which squared with his previous theories seemed to affect his organs of vision. Now this, Gentlemen, is a most pernicious though too prevalent frame of mind. When I was a little boy, I used to imagine that prejudice was a thing peculiar to some individuals. But, alas, I have since learned that we are all under its influence, and that it is only a question of degree. But let us ever contend against it, and remembering that the glorious truth is always present, let us strive patiently and humbly to discover it.

This was the fray that Koch now entered into. This was the challenge he faced: not just to prove the existence of one disease, but to change the conception of all disease.

TODAY, OF COURSE, KOCH'S WORK IS SELF-EVIDENT. WE ALL KNOW about germs. We avoid them, and we fear them. Indeed, we have so internalized the idea of germs, we so take their existence for granted, that we respond to them viscerally, with disgust. When food falls on the floor, when somebody coughs in our face or sneezes on our necks, it's revolting enough to cause some people to wretch. If anything feels like common sense to us, it is the existence of germs.

But this is entirely learned behavior. We stand today on the far end of a process that began in makeshift laboratories such as Koch's and that took decades of evidence and persuasion. Only after that process could there be a later, cultural shift—the revolution—where the existence of germs was accepted, not argued. To understand the scale of that shift is to fathom how radical an idea the germ theory was when Koch conducted his first experiments in Wöllstein.

In fact, our world today is one that has been designed meticulously around the germ theory. We live in an antiseptic culture, with Purell dispensers and masked airplane passengers and Listerine (named, of course, after the surgeon), with its promise to kill germs. These are so much part of life that we can't imagine tolerating otherwise. Even Lister might be shocked at how far our suspicion of germs has taken us.

Indeed, the pervasiveness of germophobia has given rise to mysophobia, the pathological fear of germs. This has dramatic shades of Lady Macbeth, but it also has potential scientific consequences. Our culture of mysophobes has created what is called the hygiene hypothesis, the theory among some microbiologists that we have so thoroughly rid our environment of germs that we have left ourselves too clean. In our antiseptic homes and communities, the hypothesis goes, we are no longer exposed to necessary and helpful bacteria, and our immune systems have grown weak and flabby. The result, some scientists believe, is an increase in allergies, autoimmune deficiencies, and conditions such as Crohn's disease, diabetes, and asthma.

Though the hygiene hypothesis has been around since the late 1980s, a 2012 study published in the journal *Science* offered significant support. Researchers raised mice in a sterile environment, purged of bacteria and other germs. These mice had increased allergies and intestinal colitis. But when the researchers took other, germ-free mice and exposed them to microbes during their first weeks of life, these animals developed normal immune systems.

The study was promising but, like the early work on the germ theory, mostly suggestive. The hygiene hypothesis remains just that, a hypothesis, and an especially difficult one to prove definitively at that, considering it would require humans to live in isolated environments over the span of many years. Nonetheless, the very existence of the hygiene hypothesis demonstrates how far our relationship with germs has evolved in just 130 years and how profound was the revolution that Koch and Pasteur and the rest incited.

But in April 1876, science was still on the other side of history, still wandering in a pre-germ present. Unlike everything that had come before, Koch's work on anthrax had the potential to constitute a new revolution, to compel a new conception of reality. He offered, to use Kuhn's terminology, the paradigm shift that would push normal science to a crisis.

From today's vantage point, what was happening in 1876 looks like the inexorable march of progress. Koch, sitting alone at night, hunched over his field mice and microscopes, resembles a character in the first act of a movie: the not-yet-discovered hero who, though he might be ignorant of what's in store for him, is plainly destined for greatness and glory. Moreover, lined up alongside Pasteur and Henle and the rest, Koch stands among the vanguard in a bold march toward a new, inevitable truth.

But it's important that we try, as much as we can, amid our anti-bacterial soaps and antiviral Kleenex, to recognize that these early champions of the germ theory did their work in isolation, and they faced routine resistance and outright rejection. History is inevitable, but progress is not. As Darwin's work demonstrated, nature has many dead ends, and not all development is improvement. The evolutionary biologist and scientific historian Stephen Jay Gould made this point elegantly, arguing that "great ideas, like species, do not have 'eureka' moments of sudden formulation in all their subtle complexity; rather, they ooze into existence along tortuous paths lined with blind alleys." Today's realities, in other words, were not foreordained by yesterday;

they were the result of small changes and shifts that happened to lead this way.

In April 1876, Koch took out his notebooks once more and checked his work. He had scoured the data dozens of times, double-checking his figures, testing his conclusions, probing for a mistake somewhere along the way. He needed to be certain, absolutely certain. At last he closed the notebooks. He knew this was real; he was sure of it. Though his tools were rudimentary, almost primitive, his methods were sound, his evidence thorough, and his conclusions reasonable. He had discovered something true, something that, as far as he could tell, nobody had ever discovered before. Now he just needed to tell someone.

Over the next few days, Koch dutifully treated his patients for their sprained ankles and headaches, but inside, he had drifted far away from Wöllstein. He needed to bring his conclusions . . . somewhere. But where? How?

In Wöllstein, he was far removed from any scientists or even other physicians; his closest friend may have been the Baron von Unruhe-Bomst. There were, of course, his teachers at Göttingen, including Henle. He had also studied with Hermann Lotze, a logician who pioneered the field of scientific philosophy; Lotze would certainly appreciate the rigor of Koch's work. There were other acquaintances. There was Virchow in Berlin, though he was surely too busy. In the fall of 1875, just prior to his breakthrough work on anthrax, Koch had visited the laboratory of the famous hygienist Max von Pettenkofer in Munich. But von Pettenkofer was a germ theory skeptic and represented the authority and the argument that Koch was up against in making his claim.

In the end, Koch looked not back to Göttingen, but east to Breslau—known today as Wrocław, the second-largest city in Poland.

Breslau was an established center of science, and one that was philosophically aligned with Koch's work. The University of Breslau was
home of the Institute of Plant Physiology, run by Ferdinand Cohn, an
esteemed botanist who had spent the previous decade studying bacteria. (To justify the research at his institute, he first had to establish
that bacteria were plants, not animals; they are now recognized as
neither.) Koch had been closely reading Cohn's journal, *Beiträge zur
Biologie der Pflanzen* ("Contributions to the Biology of Plants"), where
he had been publishing a series of papers under the heading "Studies
of Bacteria." In 1872, Cohn published a monograph titled "Bacteria:
The Smallest Living Organisms," in which he made an audacious
declaration:

> In recent times, our knowledge of the effects which bacteria
> can have over the life and death of humans has been
> revealed. . . . All epidemics, cholera, pestilence, typhus, diph-
> theria, variola, scarlet fever, hospital gangrene, epizootic, and
> the like, have certain features in common. These diseases do
> not arise de novo, but are introduced from another place
> where they have been prevalent, by means of a diseased person
> or through material which has been in contact with such:
> they spread only through contagion.

Koch read Cohn's words and clearly thought he had found a
comrade in arms. On April 22, 1876, he wrote to Cohn:

> Honored Professor!
>   I have found your work on bacteria, published in the
> *Beiträge zur Biologie der Pflanzen*, very exciting. I have
> been working for some time on the contagion of anthrax.
> After many futile attempts I have finally succeeded in
> discovering the complete life cycle of Bacillus anthracis. I
> am certain, now, as a result of a large number of

experiments, that my conclusions are correct. However, before I publish my work, I would like to request, honored professor, that you, as the best expert on bacteria, examine my results and give me your judgment on their validity.

Koch asked if he might visit Cohn to demonstrate his experiments. Cohn was dubious that some random country doctor might have done anything worthwhile. But he was grateful that Koch knew of his journal and invited him to Breslau the next Sunday.

Days later, Koch headed to the train station carrying microscopes, slides, cows' eyes, mouse spleens, and boxes of rabbits, frogs, and mice—many, many mice, both living and dead. Some were flush with anthrax. Rushing through the Wöllstein station to make his train, laden with his boxes and trunks, he must have been quite a sight.

At noon the next day, a Sunday, Koch knocked on the door of Cohn's home. Cohn greeted him and sent him over to the institute, where Koch began arranging his materials for the next day's demonstration. He must have been nervous. Not only would this be the first time he'd demonstrated his research, but it was surely the first time he'd worked in a professional lab since Göttingen. And now he was on the verge of revealing his kitchen-sink efforts to experts in the field.

The next morning, Koch returned to the institute and began preparing the day's experiments. He took blood from the spleen of a recently dead mouse and set up a culture in the cow's-eye humor for *Bacillus anthracis*. He also injected some precultured bacteria just under the skin of a living frog. From time to time, a few of Cohn's colleagues would stop by to check in on this unusual visitor, asking him a question or two about his work. Finally, the preparations were complete. Now he just had to wait for the bacteria to do its work. Koch met up with a friend and went to a local beer garden.

On the second day, with Cohn and several assistants watching, Koch began to go through his samples and reveal the progress. The cultured bacteria had, as he had promised, grown into a chain of rods and filaments, along with some spores as well. Cohn was particularly entranced by the appearance of spores, which he himself had recently identified in another bacteria. Fascinated, Cohn took out a notebook and sketched what he saw under the microscope. Koch did the same in his own notebook; then they compared the drawings, looking for confirmation of what their own eyes had told them. The two sets of sketches were so similar they could barely be told apart.

In what would become his trademark style, Koch was meticulous and thorough. The cultures were clean and well prepared, the observations under the microscope carefully conducted, with many redundant results. Koch's confidence grew. "My experiments were well received," he wrote in his diary that evening.

By the third day, word of Koch's experiments had spread throughout the university. Julius Cohnheim, the director of the Institute of Pathology, walked across the university grounds to visit Cohn's laboratory. A former assistant of Virchow's in Berlin and a national leader in medical science, Cohnheim was intrigued by the germ theory but not yet convinced—as such, he was a more impartial observer than Cohn. Koch showed Cohnheim his cultures and techniques, walking him through his checks and double-checks. Cohnheim followed along closely, fascinated by the work but also altogether astonished at the young man himself. He couldn't get over how methodical and thorough this Koch was; he had apparently emerged from nowhere but was calmly demonstrating the most deliberate and decisive laboratory techniques Cohnheim had ever seen.

Cohnheim complimented Koch on his scrupulous work and then left, rushing back across the campus to his pathology institute. Drop everything, he said to his assistants, and get over to Cohn's lab. You must meet Koch. "This man has made a magnificent discovery," he told them, explaining the precision with which Koch had conducted his experiments, despite the fact that he'd done it all in relative isolation. "I regard this as the greatest discovery in the field of pathology," Cohnheim said,

chasing his students out the door, "and believe that Koch will again surprise us and put us all to shame by further discoveries!"

That evening, to celebrate Koch's discovery—and to celebrate his
discovery of Koch—Cohn invited Koch to join him at his house for
dinner. Cohn's home was warm and elegant, with an ornate study
decorated with Persian rugs and all the accoutrements of a respected
nineteenth-century scientist: busts, globes, and walls of books. The
place, and the man, made a deep impression on Koch. He realized
that he had far to go, but he now had a model, and perhaps a mentor,
to guide him. Over dinner, Cohn was encouraging. Your work, he
told Koch, is tremendously promising. It must be known throughout
Europe. It might be a discovery for the ages.

Koch returned to his room that night filled with satisfaction. It
had been just a few days, barely more than a week, since he'd impetuously written to Cohn. Yet now he had shown his work and announced himself—and not only was his work considered valid, but he
was himself being taken seriously. He had been scrutinized, his work
examined, and he'd been deemed worthy. He filled his journal with a
list of people he had met: the generous Cohn; the eminent Cohnheim;
Eduard Eidam and Carl Weigert, Cohnheim's two assistants, both of
whom would turn out to be lifelong friends and allies. These were
men of science, men of stature—and now they were his fellows.

On Wednesday, Koch went back to Cohn's lab for one last day, to
finish his demonstrations for more visitors. By now Cohn was utterly
convinced. He took Koch aside and offered to publish the work in his
journal. Koch gladly accepted and returned to Wöllstein elated.

The paper, which appeared in October 1876 in Cohn's "Studies of
Bacteria" series, marked Koch's arrival from obscurity, his transition
from a country doctor dabbling with farm animals in his kitchen to a
full-fledged scientist. He quickly sent off copies to von Pettenkofer in
Munich, to Virchow in Berlin, and to the editors of the *German Medical
Journal* and the *German Quarterly for Public Hygiene*. Doing so was
telling. Though the paper had appeared in Cohn's journal, a respected

publication, that journal's subject was biological, not medical. It wasn't enough to have the work simply published; Koch wanted to be sure it found its intended audience: medical researchers as well as biologists.

The study was well received; a report in Virchow's journal, *Jahres-bericht*, wrote that Koch's was "by far the most important study on the etiology of anthrax to appear in the year." In retrospect, this is a historic understatement. In fact, Koch's paper was not merely important for one disease for one year; it was a turning point for the whole conception of disease and, even more broadly, for the natural world. Naturalists such as Darwin had brought a new understanding to the world of the connections among animals, placing every creature within the arc of creation. Now, on a microscopic scale, bacteriology was doing the same: bringing clarity of perspective and consequence to the invisible world. Koch's discovery constituted a new role for science, one that would soon go beyond the merely biological and into the new discipline of true medical science.

Koch's anthrax paper wasn't, in itself, enough to make the germ theory triumph all at once. Virchow, in particular, was unconvinced, curtly dismissing Koch's work as irrelevant to the understanding of disease. As he told Koch soon after when the latter visited Berlin, he had read the paper and still thought the "whole business seemed quite improbable." But such doubts revealed more about Virchow's recalcitrance than about Koch's work. Taken on its merits, the research was unassailable, definitive, and like nothing to have appeared before. Koch's paper was a seismic shift, an introduction of new information of such persuasiveness that it couldn't be ignored.

ALAS, IF KOCH EXPECTED THE PUBLICATION OF HIS ANTHRAX PAPER to vault him to Europe's greatest stage, he was soon enlightened. The world took notice of his work, to be sure, but the gatekeepers of science didn't swing open the gates just because he had drawn nice pictures of things he'd seen under his microscope. Back in Wöllstein, as before, Koch had patients to attend to, and they didn't care a ⸝ about bacteriology. He had a wife and daughter to provide for, and he had a hodgepodge of a laboratory, filled with second-rate equipment, do-it-yourself contraptions, and barn-bred mice.

As the months went by, and other papers followed his paper, he could see his work eclipsed. Feeling a bit sorry for himself, he wrote to Cohn: "I see from your letter that recently many new things have been reported which I, in my isolated corner of Germany, know nothing about. Well, there is nothing for it but I must come to Breslau on a visit and learn at first hand of all these exciting things."

Koch did visit Cohn in Breslau again, several times, and he'd soon publish other research in Cohn's journal. But the connection was peripheral rather than official, and Koch's visits were at Cohn's convenience; after all, Cohn and his assistants had official duties and their own research to attend to. Koch remained, he realized, fairly on his own in Wöllstein. He had connections now, but he still had to make his own way.

His next area for research, then, was especially significant. Rather than continue to study anthrax or move to another infectious disease, he instead pursued technological innovations rather than scientific discovery. In particular, he wanted to make it easier to prove the existence of bacteria by making it easier to document their existence—and he wanted to do it with photography.

Like other scientists of the time, Koch had to sketch his observations. He was a perfectionist, and although a reasonably good draftsman himself, he realized that the use of drawings allowed skeptics to quibble about whether a scientist's representation was real or accurate. The scientist was forced to be more than a witness to nature; he became nature's representative. So, to make the case, to really prove the point that germs exist as causal agents, Koch knew that hand drawings must be replaced by photographs. The only trouble was that the technology didn't yet exist that would capture images at that tiny scale.

invention of photography in the early 1800s, scientists
the first to adopt it for their own purposes. In 1840 the
sician Alfred Donné photographed sections of bone and
red blood cells. (He called his instrument the microscope-
daguerreotype.) This resolution, on the level of cells and tissue, suited
pathologists, who needed to show tumor or organ cells. But the
cameras didn't yet have a resolution capable of capturing the filaments
and flagellations of bacteria.

With characteristic initiative, Koch decided to invent a tool for
his own purposes. With photomicrographs, he explained to Cohn in
1876, he could reveal the bacteria "true to nature and free of subjective
misinterpretation."

Koch had his work cut out for him. Photography at the time was
still relatively primitive, involving glass plates, bulky wooden cassettes,
and silver-iodine emulsion baths. Adapting this apparatus to a microscope was a significant undertaking. Without electric lights, Koch
was dependent on sunlight for exposure, and he had to jury-rig a
series of mirrors to concentrate the sun's rays toward the microscope.
He began to correspond with other German scientists working on
photomicroscopy, including Gustav Fritsch, a professor of physiology
at the University of Berlin. (Fritsch had gained renown a few years
earlier for identifying the motor areas of the brain.) Comparing techniques and workarounds, Fritsch and Koch both made the breakthrough to turn their setups horizontally, rather than stacking them
vertically. This allowed for a much more stable apparatus, one capable
of both better resolution and better magnification.

Soon Koch was visiting the Carl Zeiss company headquarters in
Jena, Germany, to consult with its chief engineer, Ernst Abbe, on his
new invention for concentrating light more effectively. Called the
Abbe condenser, it would significantly improve the ability of scientists to illuminate their plates, and Koch was among the first to test
the technology.

By November 1877, Koch had successfully developed a technique that would allow any scientist to record his or her work with photographs. In the paper that followed (published in Cohn's journal), Koch explained his procedures—preparing and staining the bacteria, arranging the camera with the microscope—so that others could adopt his technique. His resulting images of *Bacillus anthracis* were the first-ever published microphotographs of bacteria. Writing to Fritsch, Koch tried to put the achievement in perspective: "I am well aware of how imperfect my photographic efforts have been, but I am absolutely certain that a bad photograph of a living organism is a hundred times better than a misleading or possibly inaccurate drawing."

Microphotography wasn't Koch's only innovation. Other improvements in laboratory tools were soon to follow, from new slide stains to culture media to plating techniques, many of which endure in basic lab protocols today. He wasn't waiting for science to reach him. He saw, like few other researchers at the time, where science needed to go.

With his new tools in hand, Koch was ready to return to his bacteriological experiments. For his next target, he chose a problem he had seen firsthand on the battlefields of France: wound infections. It had been six years since his return from the war, but the experience of seeing so many soldiers die, apparently from relatively minor wounds, had affected him deeply. Lister had provided measures that could mitigate these infections, but there was little experimental evidence demonstrating what, precisely, was happening in infected wounds, let alone which microbes were involved.

Koch's choice to study wound infections was telling, for several reasons. First and foremost, infection was a significant medical problem in his day, extracting a massive social cost in lives and resources. As Koch saw time and again in the war, a surgery might go perfectly well, with the patient apparently on the road to recovery, only to be followed by infection and the patient's death days later. The same thing happened in civilian hospitals all too regularly. In Parisian hospitals in 1870, the death rate after surgery was a staggering 60 percent; in London it was scarcely better at 40 percent. And despite Lister's efforts, conventional medicine was still a long way from reckoning with the issue. Surgery manuals of the 1870s and '80s still welcomed "laudable pus"—which refers to the notion, dating back to the fourteenth century, that pus was a welcome healing agent. (In fact, it's a worrisome buildup of white blood cells, agents of the body's losing fight against infection.)

Part of the challenge here was that, so far, bacteriology had only confused the issue. Though Klebs had clearly associated microorganisms with war wounds in 1872, he had regrettably accepted the prevailing theory that all bacteria were the same, part of a universal organism he called *Microsporum septicum*—a concept so all-encompassing as to be useless. Moreover, Klebs's organism could be found in and on perfectly healthy animals, including humans, inviting the same doubts that had dogged bacteriology and the germ theory prior to Koch's anthrax work: Was bacteria the cause of inflammation and disease or was it simply a coincidence of inflammation, with the disease caused by some other means?

Koch's task was not only to establish causation, but also to associate specific microbes with specific diseases. If he could answer the deeper questions of causation and provide a scientific basis for the rigorous application of hygienic procedures, then he would be serving not just his profession, but also society at large. It didn't hurt that the question of wounds and treatments had already gotten a great deal of attention from some of the most famous researchers in Europe: Lister, Davaine, and Klebs. There was scientific glory to be had here, and Koch knew it.

It's worth asking why science had yet failed to provide a satisfactory answer to such a profoundly important question. For decades, Semmelweis, Henle, Klebs, and scores of others had pointed their microscopes at the problem and had tried valiantly to prove that bacteria caused disease. The result was a bounty of suggestive research but nothing definitive, nothing that ultimately constituted proof, especially when measured by significant changes in hospital practices or a drop in death rates. There remained a chasm between what bacteriologists believed to be the case and what society could be convinced of.

The problem was that there were no consistent standards of evidence and proof—the essential tools for modern science. Today, of course, there are rigorous standards for performing valid research, an accepted and universal experimental protocol. There are clear steps for designing a medical experiment, such as the double-blind, randomized clinical trial, where neither the study subjects nor the researchers know who is getting which therapy, and with the subjects assigned their path randomly, so as not to introduce bias into the experiment. There are schools of epidemiology and biostatistics and quantitative analysis where researchers spend years learning how to conduct a valid scientific experiment. There are accepted procedures for analyzing the data collected, with confidence intervals, p-values, and widely accepted thresholds for statistical significance—a measure by which a researcher can say, "We have learned something new here."

Today's scientists take for granted that if they follow generally accepted processes of reliability (following best practices for experiment design), reproducibility (the ability of other scientists to repeat the experiment and produce similar results), and presentation of evidence (disclosing enough data so a reader can assess the evidence independently), their work will be taken as scientifically valid. Any scientist working today takes as a given that there are explicit boxes to check and a clear process for checking them.

But Koch and his contemporaries had no such standards. The scientific method then was a hodgepodge of practices, with no uniform protocols for posing a hypothesis, conducting an experiment, analyzing evidence, and presenting results. There were *techniques*, to be sure, but there were as yet no *standards*—and between the two lies the great chasm separating antiquated science from modern research.

This isn't to say there wasn't a gesture toward such universal rules. The scientific method available to Koch and others then can be traced back to Francis Bacon, in 1620, when he proposed a method for establishing causation through inductive reasoning. Not long after, Descartes, in the 1640s, advanced the cause of empiricism, the idea that science must be tested against observations. But neither provided explicit frameworks for how to design an experiment, let alone one for medicine. It wasn't until 1865, when the French physiologist Claude Bernard wrote "An Introduction to the Study of Experimental Medicine," that the first true effort to institute a formal process for gathering and assessing evidence appeared.

Amid such ambiguity, Robert Koch arrived on the scene. Koch's greatest virtue, it turned out, was to overinvestigate a problem, exhausting every possible argument opposed to his conclusions with a barrage of meticulously collected evidence. His lack of affiliation also proved an advantage, since he was subject to no particular procedural dogma. Elsewhere, every school pursued its own version of a scientific method, determined and governed by the laboratory chief: Cohn had his approach in Breslau (his insistence on a control group for Koch's anthrax experiment, for instance, would have been an unnecessary step to many), Virchow his in Berlin (he had little patience for theories without evidence, deeming Darwin's notions of evolution outside the scope of provable knowledge), Pasteur yet another approach in Paris, and so on. One researcher assessing the field in 1877 put it this way: "The various researchers have become embroiled in such contradictions that a survey of the studies in this field does not yield a single uncontested advance." He added: "There is something depressing in this admission for one who is searching for the truth."

Amid these competing protocols, Koch approached the problem of wound infections. Using rabbits and mice, he set out to study five different types of infections: gangrene, septicemia, pyemia (abscesses due to infection), erysipelas (a skin infection), and sepsis. His experiments went on for about nine months, a remarkably brief period by today's standards. But even in this short time, he was able to assemble enough evidence to clearly demonstrate that he had discovered something new. This was evident in the very title of his report: "The Etiology of Wound Infections." Though this title seems benign, or even generically scientific, *etiology* (meaning the cause of disease) was a bold term to use. Considering how the cause of wound infections had bewildered medicine for centuries and frustrated the greatest scientists of the age, and considering how little was known about the etiology of *any* disease whatsoever, this constituted a succinct and swaggering proclamation. He had established causality once again.

It wasn't a boast or hyperbole. Koch took the term seriously, and his paper proposed two essential conditions for establishing proper etiology. First, he maintained that the bacteria would have to be evident in all cases of a disease. "In order to prove that bacteria are the cause of traumatic infective diseases," he wrote, "it would be absolutely necessary to show that bacteria are present without exception and that their number and distribution are such that the symptoms of the disease are fully explained." His second condition was that the observed bacteria had to be distinct from one disease to another (a clear response to Klebs's failure to distinguish among *Microsporum septicum* a few years earlier). "The morphological characteristics of the bacteria found in pyemia, diphtheria, smallpox, and cholera are so similar that it is indeed easy to mistake them for identical forms," he wrote (though he mistakenly included smallpox, which is caused by a virus, not bacteria). "But this would mean that one could not assign any specific importance to these organisms. In this case they would be parasites of the diseases, not their cause."

The bacteria Koch had found were, foremost, the two great villains of infection, *Streptococcus* and *Staphylococcus*. Koch isn't generally credited with their discovery, in part because, though he had isolated both bacteria and identified them as agents of disease, even including images of the microbes in his paper, he curiously didn't venture to name the organisms he had found. Naming rights aside, Koch's

triumph here was larger than planting the flag of discovery on another microbe. Instead, his work on wound infections accomplished
something even more enduring, in two related respects. First, he
demonstrated unambiguously that specific bacteria cause specific infections. Second, he stipulated a set of threshold protocols for proving
causation, standards that could be used by others to make their own
demonstrations of causation.

These protocols, known as Koch's postulates, are perhaps what
Koch is best known for today. Though they wouldn't be presented formally as the postulates until 1884, they make their first appearance in
his report on wound infections. They can be summarized as follows:

1. The infectious agent must be present in every case of
    the disease.
2. The infectious agent must be extracted from a diseased
    individual, isolated from all other microorganisms,
    and grown independently in laboratory culture.
3. The infectious agent must create the same disease
    when introduced into a healthy test individual.
4. The supposed infectious agent must be extracted from
    the test individual and shown to be the same
    microorganism.

In these principles, Koch was building on the twin pillars of
German science, or *Wissenschaft*: *Vollständigkeit,* or completeness, and
Nachvollziehbarkeit, clarity of methods and results (what is today known
as reproducibility). He was, in other words, advancing a process for
creating legitimate science, a framework for bacteriology that would,
once and for all, allow it to emerge as a recognized and valid explanation for the cause of disease. This framework pertained to more
than bacteriology; it also offered a template for all modern medical
science and indeed all scientific investigation.

Koch's process—isolating a bacterium from a diseased organism, growing it, introducing it into a healthy organism, and then establishing disease once more—came as close as science could to affirming causation. This is no small feat; science today still grapples with the difference between correlation and causation, and Koch's postulates, in slightly revised form, continue to be used as criteria for valid research. The mantra of "correlation is not causation" is so pervasive in modern science as to be a cliché, but it is nonetheless commonly overlooked, as overeager researchers (or overeager chroniclers of research) make a wishful leap from a correlation between a disease and an agent and an actual causative relationship. Koch had laid the groundwork for a more rigorous science, one that could withstand the doubts, distractions, and obfuscation of his contemporaries.

The work on wound infections, though less celebrated than his work on anthrax or his later research on tuberculosis, would mark Koch's first demonstration of his greater scientific capacity: not just as a hunter of microbes, but as a pioneer of science. It would also be his last significant research in Wöllstein. By now, it had been more than three years since his work on anthrax. He was no longer practicing in isolation from true scientists. Through persistence, diligence, and skill (with some luck along the way), he had established himself in the vanguard of European bacteriology. He was now in regular correspondence with Cohn and Cohnheim; no longer following in Klebs's footsteps anonymously, he was now regularly corresponding with him and publicly debating him. Cohnheim invited Koch to give a lecture on his work in Kassel, and in 1879, Cohn put his name forward to join the University of Breslau. Koch was elated—this was the escape he'd been pining for—but there were no funds available for the position, and the appointment fell through. Koch remained in Wöllstein, increasingly frustrated, ready to jump at anything that offered a way out.

Then, in 1880, the director of the German Imperial Health Office, Heinrich Struck, made an argument to the kaiser that Germany's future depended on its scientific leadership. Chief among these sciences was bacteriology, which not only was germane to issues of public health, but seemed essential to combating disease in the colonial lands that Germany had assembled in Africa and Indonesia. Struck called for a new institute devoted to bacteriological research, to be based in Berlin, and he already had a lab director in mind: Robert Koch.

In early July 1880, the kaiser agreed; Struck could have his laboratory. On Wednesday, July 7, Struck sent Koch a telegram officially offering him the position. It was a terse dispatch that cut to the chase, asking when Koch could report for his new assignment. He would have to end his practice, move his wife and daughter, and find somewhere to stay in Berlin.

Koch replied at once: "I will be at your disposal in Berlin on 10 July."

The tenth was just three days away, and a Saturday. He wasn't even going to take the weekend off.

CHAPTER 3

1878 · The Rivalry

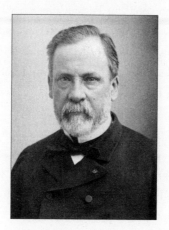

Louis Pasteur, in 1878

On April 30, 1878, a few steps away from the Seine in Paris, a man entered the grand courtyard of the Académie Nationale de Médecine. His closely cropped beard had gone white, and he walked with a limp, his left side dragging slightly, the result of a stroke nine years earlier, which made him seem much older than his fifty-five years. Slowly, carefully, the man climbed the stairs to the Session Room. This was Louis Pasteur, and he was on his way to tell the French medical establishment something few of them wished to hear.

Pasteur took the post behind the speaker's desk at the front of the chamber, a massive marble statue of Hippocrates hulking behind him. Before him were the two hundred physicians and surgeons of the academy, the most respected medical men in France. Though Pasteur belonged to the academy, he was not one of them. His training was in chemistry, and though his career was already marked by great discoveries, he was a newcomer to medicine. Many in the audience considered him an interloper. When he'd applied to the academy a few years earlier, in 1873, he'd just barely gained admission, squeaking by on a vote of 41 to 38.

Even those who voted for Pasteur's membership in the academy felt that his place was to bolster their work; instead, he quickly began challenging it. His speech of April 30, entitled "Germ Theory and Its Applications to Medicine and Surgery," would be the most provocative yet. This day, Pasteur would do nothing less than scold French medicine for putting its citizens at risk, and then school them in how they might rebuild the integrity of their profession.

Pasteur began by appealing to the academy's members as scientists. Germs, he acknowledged, were a novel idea. But science, Pasteur insisted, was a sublime process, perfectly suited to transform the unknown into the known.

> If it is terrifying to think that life may be at the mercy of the multiplication of those infinitesimally small creatures, it is also consoling to hope that Science will not always remain powerless before such enemies. . . . All is dark, obscure and open to dispute when the cause of the phenomena is not known; all is light when it is grasped.

And then he took the impudent liberty of putting himself in the surgeon's place:

> If I had the honor of being a surgeon, convinced as I am of the dangers caused by the germs of microbes scattered on the surface of every object, particularly in the hospitals, not only would I use absolutely clean instruments, but, after cleansing my hands with the greatest care . . . I would only make use of

charpie, bandages, and sponges which had previously been
raised to a heat of 130°C to 150°C.

Pasteur continued in this way for some time, explaining in detail
the precautions that surgeons should take, immediately, if they
wanted to improve their patients' chances of avoiding infection and
surviving surgery. When he finished, the audience applauded politely,
but the consternation in the room was palpable. Some were outraged,
some were convinced, and yet all of them understood that, after
Pasteur's remarks, medicine could no longer be the same. He had
issued, in effect, a declaration of war against those who clung to ideas
such as spontaneous generation or miasma. He had infiltrated their
ranks, and now he seemed dedicated to changing their profession.

Pasteur, of course, knew what he was doing. His animus toward
germs, and toward those who would deny their existence, was deeply
personal. "Do you know why it is so important to me to fight and
defeat you?" Pasteur wrote to a proponent of spontaneous generation a
few months before his "Germ Theory" speech. "It is because you are
one of the main adherents to a medical doctrine that I consider extremely harmful to the art of healing." Even for Pasteur, who'd made
his career by battling the dragons of conventional wisdom, this was
unusually blunt.

Pasteur's disdain wasn't just philosophical. He also abhorred germs
in a literal sense. In fact, he may have been history's first germophobe:
He was compulsive about washing his hands, leaving his work repeatedly throughout the day to roll up his sleeves and lather up. This
wasn't tidiness; as his nephew described later, Pasteur was convinced
that shaking hands was dangerous.

If by chance a stranger had come to call on him in the laboratory, particularly if it was a physician, and if he had been
unable to avoid this time-honored gesture of courtesy, he

gave me a slight sign that I knew well, pointing towards the sink with his head, which meant that I was to go to open the spigot.

The particular antipathy toward shaking hands with a *medical* man was telling. Those who were best served by the germ theory were also, regrettably, often the same ones who were most responsible for spreading the most dangerous germs of all—which is what compelled Pasteur to give his speech that day: Physicians were the problem, but they were also the solution. To stop them from spreading germs, Pasteur needed to convince them that there *were* germs.

Though we can't be sure when or how, sometime around his "Germ Theory" speech, Pasteur heard about Koch's breakthrough work on anthrax. Somehow, from out of nowhere, this unknown young doctor in eastern Germany had isolated the anthrax bacterium and proven, decisively, that it could be not only drawn from a diseased animal but also cultured and then inserted into another animal, which would then develop the disease. It was a remarkable feat of science, beautiful in its thoroughness, and it would have given great comfort to any champion of the germ theory. If the doubters wanted proof, here were heaps of it.

If only he hadn't been German. The thought must have crossed Pasteur's mind, for like Koch, Pasteur was very much a patriot. During the Franco-Prussian War, after German forces bombed Paris, Pasteur angrily returned an honorary degree he had received a few years earlier from the University of Bonn, Germany. "I obey a call of conscience in requesting you to erase my name from the archives of your faculty," Pasteur wrote, "and to take back this diploma as a sign of indignation which the barbarity and hypocrisy instills in a French scientist from those who, to satisfy a criminal need, insist on the massacre of two great nations."

Pasteur would bear a grudge for the rest of his life. As he once wrote to a friend after the German victory at Metz (where Koch served at the German field hospital), "each of my studies, to my dyi... day, will bear the epigraph: 'Hatred of Prussia, vengeance, vengeance!'" Sometimes this retribution took absurd form, as when he created a recipe for a special lager that, he believed, was far better than anything coming out of Munich or Berlin. He called it "Bière de la Revanche Nationale" or "the Beer of Revenge."

As word of Koch's discoveries began to spread, he began to be mentioned alongside Pasteur. This surely caught Pasteur's attention, especially when those reports cast Koch as not just a peer of Pasteur's but perhaps his successor, a younger scientist who had taken the Frenchman's broadly suggestive work and made it specifically relevant to medicine. The English physicist and essayist John Tyndall spotted this connection right away, making it in an 1876 speech on the germ theory—just months after Koch's anthrax publication: "The very first step toward the extirpation of those contagia is the knowledge of their nature; and the knowledge brought to us by Dr. Koch will render as certain the stamping out of splenic fever as the stoppage of the plague of *pébrine* by the researches of Pasteur" (*pébrine* being a disease that Pasteur had diagnosed in silkworms).

By then, Pasteur had already had a spectacularly successful career. He had made breakthroughs in three fields (chemistry, biology, and industry), discoveries that brought him great acclaim and national honors, including a Grand Prize at the 1867 World's Fair, membership in the Academy of Sciences, appointment as commander in the Legion of Honor, and an audience with Napoléon III. These laurels boosted the vanity in Pasteur, and in 1876 he tried to parlay his scientific esteem into political office. He presented himself as above partisanship, an emissary from the uncorrupted world of knowledge. "While politics with its senseless divisions saps our strength and fills our enemies with joy," he said in a campaign speech, "steam, the telegraph, and countless other miracles are transforming the world." The voters were less than convinced; in a three-way race for the local seat in the French Senate, Pasteur came in third, with just 62 votes.

cs was a diversion; his passion was the germ theory. *He*
who'd advanced it from mere theory; *he* was the one who
strated the existence of germs in the first place. Yet now
this Koch. Somehow Koch had propelled the germ theory
toward acceptance in a way that Pasteur's own discoveries never quite
had. For all his work and all his acclaim, Pasteur had never established a chain of evidence so pristine and elegant, nor one so strong
and convincing, as Koch had. This German doctor, he realized, might
have something more than luck.

Pasteur had come to the germ theory through practical, rather
than theoretical circumstances. His original inquiry into fermentation, published in 1857, came at the request of a distillery in Lille, a
city in northern France. Pasteur was a professor of chemistry at a
nearby university when the distraught father of one of his students
approached him. His distillery business, the man confessed, was
failing for some mysterious reason. Rather than getting alcohol from
his beet juice, the man told Pasteur, he was getting something like
sour milk. Pasteur began an investigation and discovered that the
juice was fermenting into lactic acid rather than alcohol. The cause, he
discerned, was a bacterium that had polluted the brew, overpowering
the yeast that would otherwise have done the work of making alcohol.
This discovery essentially invented the field of microbiology.

In 1861 he famously debunked the theory of spontaneous generation by proving, with a swan-neck flask, that germs were airborne.
And in 1865 he showed that rapidly heating wine would preserve it
from microbial spoilage, calling the process, eponymously, pasteurization.

It was in that same year that Pasteur first approached the problem
of disease—albeit disease in worms, not humans. A strange illness
had afflicted the silkworms in the South of France, threatening the
nation's silk market, an essential component of the French economy.
As the distiller had a few years before, the silk farmers appealed to
Pasteur to investigate. The disease looked, at first, like a dusting of

pepper on the worms (an attribute that gave it the name *pébrine*, a local term for "pepper").

Pasteur's first theory was that the farmers simply needed to cull their stock of silkworm eggs and select a different batch. The silk farmers followed his advice, securing a new source of eggs at tremendous cost. But the next year, the spawn was a bust, as before. Horribly embarrassed, Pasteur kept at the problem until, finally, in 1869, he fixed on the right solution. The silkworms weren't being inundated by one disease but by two, both of them bacterial. The solution, Pasteur realized, was to create a hygienic environment for them, one inhospitable for the bacteria: fresh air; dry, not damp, beds. The farmers grudgingly tried the new protocol and found that it worked. The next year's crop was larger than ever. This was landmark research, perhaps the first time that a definitive cause of disease had been identified—it was six years before Koch's work on anthrax—and it would be a model for future investigations.

Beets and silkworms might seem far removed from medical science, but in fact both represented what are known today as model organisms—nonhuman species that are thoroughly studied so that their functions might shed light on how the human organism works. Pasteur's work on fermentation, in fact, pioneered the idea of model organisms, to the extent that he was perhaps the first scientist to programmatically study yeast. Today, yeast is one of the most studied organisms on the planet and has contributed mightily to our understanding of DNA, cancer, and various biotechnologies. It was up to Pasteur, though, to suggest that what he'd learned about yeast might inform a larger understanding of other microbes and human health. As far back as 1859, he'd spotted this connection: "Everything indicates that infectious diseases owe their existence to similar causes" to fermentation.

May we not believe by analogy that the day will come when easily applied preventive measures will stop the scourges

whose sudden appearance devastates and terrifies entire populations, such as the yellow fever that has recently invaded
Senegal and the Mississippi Valley or the plague that has
raged on the banks of the Volga?

Though Pasteur may have sensed the connection between human
disease and the microbial world he was exploring, it would be years
before he followed up the observation with real research.

Perhaps he was gun-shy. After all, Pasteur's first foray into human
disease, back in 1865, hadn't gone well. That year, a cholera epidemic
broke out in Marseille and Paris, France's two largest cities. Pasteur was
recruited to lead the investigation. He searched for a germ he could
identify, but in the wrong place: He examined the air in hospital wards
rather than the blood in the victims' cadavers. Maybe he was too willing
to accept the miasma theory; maybe he wasn't yet able to grasp the
awesome implications of his own discoveries—that these germs he had
discovered didn't lurk just in beer and wine, but in human bodies, too.
Whatever the reason, the cholera investigation was fruitless, and
Pasteur soon retreated to his work on wine and silkworms.

Eventually, though, medicine found him. In the 1860s, Joseph
Lister was practicing surgery at the Glasgow Royal Infirmary. After
reading Pasteur's descriptions of fermenting cheeses and putrefied
meat, Lister went to his hospital and caught a whiff of an infected
wound alive with pus and the smell of putrefied flesh. The smell, he
realized, was just as Pasteur had described it. Perhaps, Lister thought,
this might be the smell of rotting flesh. (These days, that particular
odor is foreign to our noses, but it wasn't so uncommon in the time
before refrigeration and pasteurization. Indeed, once it smacks your
nasal passages, the odor is unforgettable.) Since Pasteur's work had
clearly argued that microbes caused this rot, Lister took the next step
and proposed that, as with meat, so with wounds. Then he went a step
further: If wounds *did* teem with microbes, then purging them with a

bath of carbolic liquid or, later, a spray might eliminate infection from the start.

Lister began to experiment with antiseptic methods in his operating room, publishing his remarkable results in *The Lancet* in 1867. Seven years later, in 1874, Lister finally mustered the courage to write Pasteur directly. Praising his "brilliant researches," he told Pasteur that his discoveries had "furnished me with the principle upon which alone the antiseptic system can be carried out." Writing back, Pasteur confessed that he was "rather uninformed" about Lister's work—an astonishing admission given how decisive Lister's prescriptions had been to the German success in the Franco-Prussian War and how they would seem to offer Pasteur some practical evidence for the germ theory. But Pasteur was savvy enough to politely return the favor, complimenting Lister on the "precision of your manipulations, and by your perfect understanding of the experimental method."

By 1878, Pasteur recognized that if medicine would not heed his advice and change from within, then he must muster the evidence and change it from without. The implications of the germ theory for medicine were too great, he realized, and the stakes (in human life) too grave, to ignore the opportunity any longer.

Then came this curious news of Koch's experiments in rural Germany, and Pasteur quickly decided upon a disease for his next investigation: anthrax. Though it hadn't been a subject of his research previously, anthrax made certain sense as a subject for him. After all, he was often guided by economic implications, and anthrax was of great cost and concern to agriculture, in France as in Germany. It was also clearly the work of microbes, as Koch had shown. What's more, it was a disease that, unlike the silkworm parasites, sometimes crossed over into humans. Finally, it was a matter of pressing national interest; just months earlier, an outbreak of anthrax had run riot through the French department of Eure-et-Loir. So when Pasteur had another request, this time from the French minister of agriculture, asking him to investigate the disease, the answer was clear. How could a patriot refuse?

He got to work right away. He began by culturing the bacteria, as Koch had; he took a sample of blood from an animal that had died of anthrax, diluted it in urine (used because of its sterility), then took a sample of the mixture and placed it in a second flask of urine. He repeated this process again and again, until, as his former assistant and first biographer Émile Duclaux described later, "the original drop of blood, the one that furnished the first seed, has been drowned in an ocean. . . . Only the bacterium has escaped dilution, for it multiplies in each one of the cultures." Pasteur then injected a rabbit with a drop taken from the last flask. When the rabbit died, Pasteur had ably replicated Koch's experiment and had proven to himself that the anthrax bacterium caused the disease.

News of Pasteur's research soon made its way to Koch in Wöllstein. Koch agonized over the idea that the French giant was tackling the same terrain he had. Just months ago, nobody in the world seemed to care about anthrax, but now here was the most famous scientist in Europe, the man who had forced the germ theory from the impossible to the probable, working on the same microbe. But, if Koch felt threatened, there was little he could do about it. In a letter to Cohn back in Breslau, Koch mentioned that he'd read a translation of Pasteur's experiment and found it "very interesting," he granted. "If I only could study Pasteur's work in the original French."

His anxiety was surely made worse by the fact that Pasteur seemed entirely ignorant, perhaps willfully so, of Koch's work. Indeed, it was as if Koch had never existed to Pasteur. In these first publications on anthrax, Pasteur referred to the anthrax bacteria as *bacteridia,* using the term coined by his countryman Davaine in 1863, rather than Koch's term, *Bacillus anthracis.* (In a footnote, Pasteur did make a passing reference to Koch's work by referring to the *"Bacillus anthracis* of the Germans.")

In his next experiments, though, Pasteur demonstrated how his pragmatic approach might be more profoundly useful than Koch's laboratory work. In particular, he wondered about the mystery of anthrax's "champs maudits," or "cursed fields." Upon these fields, entire flocks of livestock might die of the disease in one season. Then the disease would disappear for years, only to return and unleash its terror once again. If bacteria caused the disease, Pasteur wondered, what happened to them in those intervening years? Where did they go— and why did they later come back?

To solve the mystery, Pasteur began searching for anthrax's hiding place, somewhere in the natural environment. He found it almost in plain sight: in the soil itself. When the animals died en masse, farmers would routinely bury them in a pit, dug in the same fields where they dropped. Some carcasses, inevitably, would be less than a meter below the surface. That was deep enough to keep the bacteria away for several years. But over time, the lowly earthworm would make its way through the carcasses and slowly nudge the microbes and their spores back up toward the surface, where they would at last attach to the next season's grass. Then a sheep or cow eating thistle or sharp grass might get a little dirt in its mouth. The thistle or grass would inflict tiny cuts in the animal's mouth, and the spores would opportunistically enter the body.

It was a brilliant bit of sleuthing on Pasteur's part, as rationally thorough as Koch's research in the anthrax life cycle had been. Pasteur's work gave vision to a different life cycle of the disease, on a human, rather than bacteriological, scale. His finding had significant implications for farmers. He laid down the law for them: "You must prevent your animals from grazing in pastures where dead bodies have been buried. Fields where crops are grown must not be used as cemeteries. Grazing or raising forage must not take place on land where dead bodies are buried."

Pasteur wasn't satisfied, though, with trodding on the familiar ground of causality. By this time he thought he understood how anthrax worked—how it lived and how it killed. This gave him an advantage, he thought; perhaps he could turn the microbe against itself. Maybe he could create a way to stop it.

In 1879 he began a side project on chicken cholera, a persistent bane of the French poultry farmer. He had successfully isolated the bacterium and was tinkering with various cultures of it. One day, by chance, he noticed that some cultures, though clearly identifiable as the chicken cholera microbe, didn't actually produce disease in birds. The microbes seemed to have lost their potency. This might have been merely frustrating, if Pasteur hadn't recalled the work of Edward Jenner, nearly a century before, on smallpox.

In 1796, Jenner, a well-respected doctor in southern England, observed that milkmaids often came down with cowpox, a debilitating but usually mild illness, apparently as a result of their work. He subsequently observed that those maids who'd had cowpox rarely contracted smallpox, a far more serious but similar disease. At the time, it was already known that people could be immunized against smallpox with an injection of a bit of tissue from somebody with the disease, a process known as variolation. But this was a dangerous practice, as a not-insignificant number of people so immunized actually came down with the disease and died, and thus variolation was far from widespread.

The milkmaids' immunity, though, suggested an experiment. Jenner took some pus from a blister on the hands of a maid named Sarah Nelmes and injected it into the arms of eight-year-old James Phipps, the son of Jenner's gardener. The boy came down with a fever but quickly recovered. Then came another experiment, one that was purely the logical next step but that was also so dangerous that no medical board would have tolerated it today: Jenner took live smallpox and injected the boy (just eight years old!) with it. Nothing happened. He tried again, and still young Phipps was fine. It was a remarkable discovery: a safe way to protect people from a disease.

Jenner's new process (later known as vaccination, from the Latin root *vaca*, for "cow") would soon become widespread. In time, many European countries adopted it into law, and it ultimately has saved millions of lives worldwide. For eighty years, Jenner's feat would be unequaled. (Smallpox would be eliminated from the face of the earth in 1973, the first and, as of now, still the only disease to be entirely eradicated from the human population.)

Pasteur had Jenner's breakthrough in mind when he noticed his weakened bacteria. With an inkling of what might happen next, he injected the weakened microbe into several birds, waited a few days, and then injected the birds again with a fresh, pure sample of active chicken cholera. The birds survived, just as Pasteur had hoped they might. They had been vaccinated, protected against disease.

This was terrific news for chicken farmers, and a few years earlier, it might have satisfied Pasteur as well. But this time Pasteur decided to repeat the experiment on animals with anthrax. For a few months, he worked in his laboratory on the rue d'Ulm in Paris. In March 1881 he announced that he had devised a technique; they might attenuate the anthrax bacterium. But it needed a practical test, not in the laboratory but in the dust and fields of a farmyard. So, in April 1881, Pasteur accepted an invitation to conduct a public test of his vaccine.

The experiment took place on May 5, 1881, on a farm in the town of Pouilly-le-Fort, a village just forty-odd kilometers outside Paris. The farm was typically, beautifully French: The barn and stable were fortified with thick stone walls, and the fields and pastures rolled out amiably toward the horizon. Pasteur, who had a natural flair for spectacle, had eagerly allowed the experiment to be publicized. As a result, the farm was crowded with hundreds of spectators: farmers, politicians, veterinarians, and, most significantly, journalists. In a large pen, sixty animals (cows, sheep, and goats) were crowded together. The local Society of French Farmers had provided the animals for the experiment.

The atmosphere was noisy and festive. Amid the animals' bleating and baaing and mooing, Pasteur began his experiment. First he examined the animals, rejecting two sheep and one cow as suspiciously weak. Then he began the vaccinations, injecting a syringe of anthrax culture into twenty-four sheep, six cows, and one goat; the bacteria was living but attenuated, meaning it had been bred into a less virulent strain. He also included a control group of about the same number of animals; these were not inoculated. Thus ended the first day of the demonstration. The crowd dispersed, and Pasteur and his assistants returned to Paris.

Less than two weeks later, on May 17, the experiment resumed. Before just as large a crowd, Pasteur gave the experimental group a second injection of the vaccine. Then, on May 31, he returned and gave all the animals, including the control group, a dose of fresh, strong anthrax culture, enough to kill. The parties then agreed to meet again in forty-eight hours to observe the results.

Among the unvaccinated control animals, the disease quickly did its work. Over the next two days, animals started breathing heavily and stopped eating. Their legs buckled, and they began falling over dead. Soon bodies littered the pens, and ailing animals stepped around the carcasses of their brethren until they, too, dropped dead. By June 2 all the unvaccinated sheep and the goat were dead, and most of the unvaccinated cows were on their way there. Even to farmers, used to dead animals, it was a horrific sight.

But the vaccinated animals were just fine. There they were, grazing in the next pasture, just as they had been for the past month. These animals were healthy—thriving, even—and entirely oblivious to the carnage just a few meters away.

On the afternoon of June 2, Pasteur returned to the farm. As his carriage crested a nearby hill, he observed the field scattered with the corpses of dead livestock. At first he couldn't tell which animals—the infected or the inoculated—were lying dead. But when the crowd recognized him and broke out in cheers, he raised his arms in triumph. "Here it is!" he cried. "Oh ye of little faith!"

The news of Pasteur's anthrax vaccine itself spread like a virus throughout Europe. Fortuitously, a correspondent from the London

Times had witnessed the experiment, as had others from several agricultural journals. Their reports didn't dabble with the science; they cut to the chase with the ignorant enthusiasm of journalists: Pasteur had triumphed. He had found a vaccine for the horrible scourge anthrax.

Pasteur was elated, and for good reason. He had created the first vaccine in nearly a century, and along the way had crafted a process that connected the diagnostic value of the germ theory with a far more practical preventive purpose. As he described it at a scientific meeting in Paris a few months later, "We now possess a vaccine of anthrax which is capable of saving animals from this fatal disease; a virus vaccine that is itself never lethal; a live vaccine, one that can be cultivated at will and transported without alteration."

This was no mere scientific discovery; this was something that would save lives—not just of animals, but perhaps of people, too. If he was a celebrated scientist before, he was a champion of the people now. He had matched Jenner and, by pure brilliant sleuthing, found a way to destroy a disease before it could destroy a flock, or a town, or a country.

On July 31, 1881, with the triumph of Pouilly-le-Fort spreading through Europe, Pasteur crossed the English Channel bound for London. His destination was St. James's Palace and the Seventh International Medical Congress.

Though there had been previous grand meetings on medicine, this seventh congress promised something of historical proportion. It seemed perfectly timed to capture a new passion for the potential of science. The *British Medical Journal,* its hometown pride evident, was effusive:

> It is always possible to exaggerate the greatness of events, as it
> is of monuments, to which we are in too close a proximity. . . .
> The mere fact of the meeting together in such unprecedented

numbers of the leading powers engaged in the study and practice of medicine and the pursuit of collateral scientific work, has been a circumstance of which the influence in the future cannot but be long and deeply felt, and of which the present results are as interesting as they have been delightful.

More than three thousand scientists attended from seventy countries—from "every land in which scientific medicine is practiced," as *The Lancet* described it. The delegates were entertained as if they were dignitaries, feted by London's most prominent citizens, including the lord mayor of London and the Baroness Burdett-Coutts. Pasteur was there, to discuss his spectacular work on the anthrax vaccine, as was Koch, who spoke about some remarkable laboratory techniques he'd developed at his new quarters in Berlin. Virchow was in attendance, as was Lister, and William Osler, the Canadian physician who would go on to cofound Johns Hopkins Hospital. The congress served as a political stage as well. The Prince of Wales gaveled the first session open, and the crown prince of Russia made an appearance. (The germophobe Pasteur, to his chagrin, found himself obliged to shake hands with the prince.)

Pasteur's work on an anthrax vaccine was the big news, and he was clearly the man of the hour. When he was introduced in the immense hall, cheers rang out "not once only," described a report in *The Popular Science Monthly*, "but again and again, [for] the scientific veteran whose renown has spread from his quiet Parisian laboratory over the whole civilized world."

The enthusiasm in London was more than just scholarly. Medical sciences were fast becoming essential economic tools, partly to address the needs of Europe's crowded cities and also as a necessity for overseas colonization and empire building. As countries raced to exploit their holdings in Africa and Asia, they were confronting infectious diseases such as malaria, cholera, and sleeping sickness, illnesses that threatened both indigenous populations and the new European colonialists.

The medical congress offered an essential forum where the germ theory could be discussed and debated. The agenda, accordingly, was filled with bacteriological demonstrations and lectures. This was due largely to Lister's efforts—he had made sure that both Pasteur and Koch were in attendance. Lister was an unabashed enthusiast for the germ theory and its potential for medicine. Just a year earlier he had suggested, presciently, that "an appropriate 'vaccine' may be discovered for measles, scarlet fever, and other acute specific diseases in the human subject." And being neither French nor German, he was free to admire Koch's work as well as Pasteur's.

It turned out, in fact, that Lister had been following Koch's research closely since the latter's anthrax paper in 1876; in an address to the British Medical Association in August 1880 he had praised Koch's inspired work on anthrax and infections. "Though a hard worked general practitioner, Koch has contrived to devote an immense amount of time and energy to his investigations," Lister said. "He has succeeded in demonstrating the presence of these minute organisms in a manner never before attained."

Though Pasteur had the spotlight at the 1881 medical congress, Koch had been making his own advances in recent months (albeit of a much less theatrical variety). In particular, he had been improving his laboratory techniques, methods that would help make the germ theory more-accepted science. Koch demonstrated his advances in Lister's lab during the medical congress, and crowds packed in tight around Koch's tables and instruments. First, Koch showed his microphotography tools, explaining how he had refined the lens and isolated the bacteria in photographs. Then he turned to his latest breakthrough: a new technique for culturing bacteria. Traditionally, bacteriologists worked with liquid organic materials such as milk or, in Koch's ingenious case, the optical fluid from inside a cow's eye.

Bacteria flourished in these environments, but liquid was a difficult medium to work with. The microbes moved about in the fluid and could be impossible to isolate, making it difficult to measure their growth.

He had noticed, though, that bacteria and molds readily grew upon a cooked potato—and that, moreover, they would grow outward from their point of origin. This made it far easier to isolate the microbes and accurately measure them. But germ cultures grew inconsistently on potato slices, keeping Koch on the lookout. He soon discovered that gelatin was much more promising, especially since it could be poured evenly on a glass plate.

The advance here was purely technical; it offered a better method for pursuing science. But this makes his breakthrough no less significant. The paper Koch published explaining his work, which he blandly titled "Methods for the Study of Pathogenic Organisms," is still referred to today as the bible of bacteriology. As with his work on microphotographs and on wound infections, the methods he detailed in the paper gave the germ theory a scientific rigor and a process that it had lacked previously.

Demonstrating these techniques in Lister's lab in London, Koch displayed a distinct lack of showmanship. Keeping his head down and speaking almost in a mumble, he quietly explained his methods, his manner the antithesis of Pasteur's razzle-dazzle performances. To those not paying close attention, his presentation would have seemed a mundane recitation of banal laboratory procedures. But his demeanor was deceptive. With each gesture, each tool, Koch was pushing science forward and giving other scientists a platform for further progress. Among those in the audience was Louis Pasteur, who couldn't help but be impressed. As Koch finished his demonstration and the observers began leaving the room, Pasteur stepped over to him. "C'est un grand progrès, Monsieur," he said.

In the weeks following the congress, Koch and his assistants would improve the plating technique considerably. After one assistant,

Walther Hesse, told his wife about the gelatin technique and mentioned that it wasn't yet perfect—the gelatin tended to turn runny in hot weather—she suggested they try agar, a similar but stabler substance derived from seaweed that she used to make jelly. It worked splendidly—so much so that it continues to be the standard medium for most cultures today. The invention was soon improved upon by another assistant in Koch's lab, Julius Richard Petri, who replaced the flat glass plates that Koch had been using with round plates with raised edges. This, of course, was the petri dish, the very plate that continues to be used to this day in laboratories the world over.

THE PROCESS OF EXPLORING, PROVING, AND REPLICATING SCIENTIFIC discoveries is, in the twenty-first century, a highly regimented one. Science journals have clear standards of evidence, require several rounds of peer review before publication, and demand that enough data be provided so that other scientists might replicate the experiment, in the hope of replicating the result. In turn, the journals themselves are assessed for their significance and impact—what's known as impact factor, a measure of how much authority a scientific journal holds in its field. The more frequently a journal's publications are cited, the higher that journal's impact factor. This network of citations and ideas and publications is the informing framework for contemporary science. It allows scientists to get their work published and to obtain funding for further research.

Though the process has its faults (belabored and inattentive peer review, exorbitantly expensive journals whose articles are inaccessible to the general public, delays of two or three years between an experiment's conclusion and its publication), without it, modern science could not happen. It is a remarkably effective system for turning questions into conclusions, and an efficient way to measure the value of science and to reward scientists (through recognition and stature and funding) to do more of it.

But in 1881, this system did not yet exist. An increasing number of scientific journals were being published, many of them, such as *The Lancet* and *Nature* in England and *Comptes rendus* in France, related to the biological and medical sciences. Even then, citations were a recognized part of the process, both putting one's own work in context and attributing credit to others. But other parts of today's system—external peer review, for instance—had yet to be established. On the pro side, this allowed science to go from laboratory to publication with remarkable speed; only the editor served as a gatekeeper. Koch's wound infections paper, for instance, was published just three weeks after he finished it. On the con side, the landscape of publications looked something of a mess, with few checks on research methods and protocols besides the opinion of that one journal editor.

An essential part of this system, then as now, is competition. The base human instinct to beat the other guy is an essential characteristic of science, notwithstanding its tweedy reputation. Without competition, there would be no need for a citation—the coin of the realm for scientists. Without competition, there would be no triumph of discovery, no glory in being first to discern a truth where there had been only questions. Economists have long recognized the essential role of competition in fostering innovation and as a spur toward technological innovation. Competition pushes innovators and companies to develop better products in order both to grow and to dominate markets. Competition makes things happen.

Which brings us back to Koch and Pasteur. While there were undoubtedly any number of practical reasons for Pasteur to turn to anthrax in 1878, including that local outbreak of the disease in rural France, the idea of besting a German scientist likely spurred him on. And now that Pasteur had made such a breakthrough, Koch was clearly game to fight back. Though the progress toward a vaccine went far beyond what he'd been able to achieve, it's clear that Koch saw Pasteur's anthrax work as a challenge to his own research on the disease. And he seemed more inclined to defend his turf in return than to give Pasteur his due.

To put it bluntly: Koch came out swinging. A few months after the London meeting, working with his two assistants Georg Gaffky and Friedrich Loeffler, he published a scathing attack on Pasteur's experimental methods and his conclusions. The world may have hailed Pouilly-le-Fort as a breakthrough for humankind, but Koch wasn't having it. "Of these conclusions of Pasteur on the etiology of anthrax, there is little which is new, and that which is new is erroneous," Koch wrote. "Up to now, Pasteur's work on anthrax has led to nothing."

Koch challenged the work on every front. He assailed Pasteur's earthworm hypothesis, casting doubt on whether earthworms could really be a vector for the disease in soil.

The theory on the role of the earthworm in the etiology of anthrax, even as with earlier investigations of Pasteur turned out to be in error; and all the proofs from his anthrax studies allow one to summarize that up to now thanks to Pasteur our knowledge of anthrax has not been enlarged; thus in part his work in this field only confuses what is already fixed or is fast being clarified.

Koch based his criticisms partly on the critical test of reproducibility—Koch had tried and failed to grow the anthrax bacteria at the temperature Pasteur claimed to have done so—but his tone was hyperbolic, crass, and altogether unbecoming. He lashed out at Pasteur with almost casual cruelty. It was quite unlike the self-deprecating fastidiousness of the letter he'd written to Ferdinand Cohn just six years earlier. Was he offended that Pasteur had outdone him? Peeved that his own dominion over anthrax was so short-lived? Whatever the perceived injustice that drove him, Koch threw the growing heft of his reputation at Pasteur's work. If Koch wanted to measure how much clout he had built up in science, he chose an especially nasty way to evaluate it.

Koch's attack was reprinted in French in February 1882, and the French scientific world was taken aback. Pasteur quickly sent his assistant Louis Thuillier to Berlin, for the stated purpose of demonstrating the vaccine, but also to allow Pasteur to gather some intelligence on his German rival. Thuillier's report, full of French condescension, didn't reflect well on any of them:

> M. Koch is not liked by his colleagues. M. Struck [the German official who had given Koch his appointment] is an intriguing ignoramus who has obtained his position as director of the Reichsgesundheitsamt only because he is von Bismarck's physician. He is very unpopular and his protege, M. Koch, shares some of the contempt in which his protector is held. Furthermore, having always lived in a small town of Posen, far away from the scientific centers, [Koch] is a bit of a rustic, and is ignorant of parliamentary language.

After an initial too-potent dose of vaccine proved toxic to German cows, Thuillier's experiments were a success. Nonetheless, Koch remained personally unconvinced and publicly unapologetic.

Pasteur himself kept silent until the next September, when he appeared at the International Congress of Hygiene and Demography in Geneva, Switzerland. With Koch sitting in the front row, Pasteur went through the history of his anthrax vaccine, back to the experiments with chicken cholera four years prior. He explained the results of his repeated experiments in Pouilly-le-Fort and subsequent sites. "Yet however blazingly clear the demonstrated truth," Pasteur remarked, "it has not always had the privilege of being easily accepted. I have encountered, both in France and abroad, obstinate objectors." In case that wasn't overt enough, Pasteur implicated Koch outright, referring to the latter's published critiques. "Dr. Koch . . . finds nothing remarkable in this experiment. . . . The author does not believe that I operated as I said I did." The clear impression was that with all the evidence Pasteur had assembled, Koch was simply in denial.

This was as close as science could get to an outright duel. Pasteur had taken his shot and, by all accounts, scored a hit, with Koch right there in the first row. Moments later, Koch was invited to the lectern for a response. He didn't hesitate to swat back.

> When I saw in the program of the Congress that M. Pasteur was to speak today on the attenuation of virus, I attended the meeting eagerly, hoping to learn something new about this very interesting subject. I must confess that I have been disappointed, as there is nothing new in the speech which M. Pasteur has just made. I do not believe it would be useful to respond here to the attacks which M. Pasteur has made on me, for two reasons: first, because the points of disagreement between Pasteur and myself relate only indirectly to the subject of hygiene, and second because I do not speak French well and M. Pasteur does not speak German at all, so that we are unable to engage in a fruitful discussion. I will reserve my response for the pages of the medical journals.

Pasteur quickly retorted that had Koch been able to follow his lecture, he would have easily grasped the new evidence presented. But, he added, he would happily wait for Koch to compose his response in print. Privately, meanwhile, Pasteur wrote with glee to a colleague that "Koch acted ridiculous and made a fool of himself." He wrote to his son, the former soldier, "It was a triumph for France; that is all I wanted."

Koch's reply, published a few weeks later, was an outrageous outburst: ten thousand words of insults, abuse, and condescension. It's worth quoting one long passage, if only to get an earful of Koch's venom:

> Concerning inoculation against anthrax, all that we heard was some completely useless data about how many thousands of animals had been inoculated. . . . All this material served solely as a vehicle for a violent polemic directed against me. . . . Thus, because of the lack of microscopic investigation, because of the use of impure substances, and because he used unsuitable test animals, Pasteur's method must be rejected as defective. . . .
>
> His biases got the better of him, and he reported wonderful things about the diseases found in his test animals and about the remains in their corpses. After all, Pasteur is not a physician, and one cannot expect him to make sound judgments about pathological processes and the symptoms of diseases. By so much the more, therefore, were his medical associates obliged to warn him against the grossest errors. . . .
>
> Pasteur deserves criticism not only for his defective methods, but also for the way in which he has publicized his investigations. In industry it may be permissible or even necessary to keep secret the procedures that lead to a discovery. However, in science different customs prevail. Anyone who expects to be accepted in the scientific community must publish his methods, so that everyone is able to test the accuracy of his claims. Pasteur has not met this obligation. . . .
>
> Thus, Pasteur follows the tactic of communicating only favorable aspects of his experiments, and of ignoring even decisive unfavorable results. Such behavior may be appropriate for commercial advertising, but in science it must be totally rejected. At the beginning of his Geneva lecture, Pasteur placed the words "Nous avons tous une passion supérieure, la passion de vérité." [We all have a greater passion, a passion

for truth.] Pasteur's tactics cannot be reconciled with these words. His behavior is simply inexplicable.

On and on it goes like this, for page after page. Koch interspersed his derisive volleys with dismissive critiques of Pasteur's methods. Repeatedly, Koch claims to be championing proper scientific procedures, and every time, he places Pasteur as being outside this method. He even tossed in what he regarded as the worst insult of all: "Pasteur is not a physician." By this time, the entire European community of medical scientists was reading, agog, the testy battle between these two titans of science. And it was only going to get worse.

Pasteur composed his response, an open letter, published in the *Revue scientifique* on Christmas Day 1882, a fact that shows how deeply the attacks affected the French scientist. This time, Pasteur uncorked his sense of outrage and let it spew. "You ascribe to me errors that I have not committed," he cried; "you denounce them and make a lot of noise with your triumph. . . . You are wrong, sir, you are setting yourself up for another foiled expectation in which you will be forced to change your opinion." And so the Frenchman railed on against the German, giving as well as he got.

The feud between Pasteur and Koch is one of the great battles of science, in part because they were so foolishly public with it. But behind the quarrels over the science itself, there have been few explanations for the rancor and its pointedly personal nature. Many historians, understandably, have attributed the whole thing to French-German antagonism, citing Pasteur's remarks in letters and Koch's appeals for German diligence. Undoubtedly, the two were both patriots and relished the chance to take on a fight with national significance. There's reason to believe part of the initial antagonism was sparked through simple miscommunication. In his remarks in Geneva, Pasteur evidently referred to Koch's published work as "recueil allemand," meaning "collection of German works." But Koch's translator in the front row heard this as "orgueil allemand"—"German arrogance."

Hearing this mistranslation, Koch felt personally insulted and reacted in kind. (Ironically, his reaction was a perfect display of what may be described as German arrogance.) Pasteur, of course, had no way of knowing that his words had been erroneously transformed into an insult, so he was rightly shocked when what he considered a scientific debate turned personally ugly.

But patriotism was only part of what was going on. Reading the petulant dialogue closely, one sees that, at root, theirs was a debate over an issue that has long turned respected scientists into petulant sticklers: the matter of credit and recognition for one's work. Pasteur and Koch were each aggrieved that the other had denied him the equivalent of a citation—a footnote or a reference or some indication that the one recognized the other's work.

In the middle of Koch's critique, he includes this:

Pasteur believes that he has discovered the etiology of anthrax. This etiology could only be established by identifying the enduring forms of anthrax bacilli, the conditions of their origin, their characteristics, and their relation to soil and water. Although I have no interest in priority disputes, these matters are so obvious that I cannot ignore them. I can only answer Pasteur's claims by referring to my publication of 1876 that describes the generation of anthrax spores and their relation to the etiology of anthrax. Pasteur's first work on anthrax was published one year later, in 1877. This requires no further comment.

Reading this, Pasteur obviously spotted a sore spot for Koch, and he picked at the scab accordingly. First, Pasteur pointed out that he had, in fact, been among the first scientists outside Germany to give Koch a public nod—which he had, not in the 1877 original paper, but in a speech that same year before the Academy of Sciences in Paris, where he described Koch's anthrax paper as "a remarkable memoir."

But then Pasteur throws the same offense back at Koch, noting that Koch's etiology of anthrax bore a great debt to Pasteur's own work with silkworms.

Why did you hide all of this to the readers of your first memoir? Are you going to say that you have ignored the existence of my work on the diseases of the silk worm, which was published in 1869–70? Your assertion would be insignificant because, in matters of science, no one is permitted to ignore a discovery, and moreover, how many opportunities did you not have, since 1877, to come back on these facts! . . . In one word, sir, it is not you who has made the discovery of the mode of generation of the bacilli, and the vibrio spoors; it is not you who has brought attention to their curious mode of formation; it is not you who has recognized their preservation in dust form and the long duration of their vitality. The precision with which I have described the formation of these ganglia, corpuscular-germs, and spoors, is such that you could have resorted simply to making a copy of the figure which illustrates this on page 228 of my work in order to introduce it in your memoir of 1876, and make use of it to illustrate what you have said about the *bacillus anthracis*.

Their mutual spite, it turns out, was based on their mutual impression that their landmark work had been not just slighted, but also deliberately ignored. Each felt that his greatest rival had not had the respect to give him his proper due. To men such as Koch and Pasteur, who were so aware of the portentous nature of their discoveries, this wasn't just an insult; it was an attempt to write the other out of history. They may have been enlisted in a common fight for the germ theory, and against all that passed as science before the germ theory, but that larger fellowship was overshadowed by pique. Without the public recognition of one for the other, there was no room for magnanimity; each could only take umbrage at the insult.

If there's a silver lining here, it's that each plainly cared about the opinion of the other—and was hurt when his rival didn't note how his work was drawing on the other's. It's unfortunate as well because both were in favor of standards for science, and it was both of them, together, who were advancing the cause of science. Building on each other's work, building on each other's discoveries, pushing for the reproducibility of the results—this is how science is supposed to happen. Even their argument itself, as public and hostile as it was, demonstrated that science was shifting toward clearer standards and protocols. Their mistake was to make that process so personal and for each to search so vigorously for the other's failures rather than recognize his merits. The sight of these two great visionaries sullying themselves may have made for great theater, but it was surely embarrassing to two men who, otherwise, stood as champions of reason over emotion.

So who was right? From our vantage point today, we can see that while Koch may have been right about a detail or two in Pasteur's process, he was altogether wrong to castigate Pasteur's work as a whole. Koch may have resented Pasteur's theatrical methods or his experimental élan, but Pasteur's instincts had rightly guided him to a valid conclusion about the role of earthworms and about the viability of the vaccine. The keen powers of observation that had served Koch so well previously—as when he assessed wound infections in Wöllstein or when he recognized that a simple potato could be a transformative medium for cultures—had failed him this time. The cool demeanor that had allowed his every success had been, at least in this exchange, abandoned. In its place were pique and anger and unseemly ruthlessness. Koch was too quick to light wildfires where candles would have been more appropriate—and it wouldn't be the last time.

BACK IN BERLIN, THE ROUTINE WORK IN KOCH'S NEW LAB WAS thankfully far removed from the drama of open letters and public denunciations. In this small warren of rooms, with the stench of caged animals and the acrid pinch of chemicals filling the air, the day-to-day lab work would have been nearly overwhelming, leavened only by the discoveries that the work so steadily yielded.

For Koch in particular, the daily work was all-consuming. Gaffky and Loeffler, two lab assistants he'd been assigned when he arrived in 1880, were soon joined by two more assistants, and then still others. Koch's work started to gain official attention, and accordingly, his resources grew. This was surely a mixed blessing, not just because of the effort it took to manage a growing laboratory. He was completely untrained for such a role and, apart from his days in university at Göttingen, hadn't spent much time even with other scientists. In the space of a few months, he went from being a solo scientist, with his own procedures and habits, to working in a busy laboratory filled with assistants. Koch had to determine quickly not only how to perform science in this new milieu, but also how to lead others, teach them his methods, and externalize what had been, for years, a strictly internal process.

To his credit, he seemed to handle it. Within the first year in Berlin, his staff published a half dozen breakthrough papers on their bacteriological discoveries. Koch himself published at least three major papers, including one on plating techniques and cultures, another on disinfection. The disinfection paper was notable because it was one of the first rigorous analyses of Lister's carbolic acid and how it worked. Koch found that, in fact, carbolic acid didn't kill all microbes, leaving some room for improvement. So Koch explored different combinations of boric acid, hydrochloric acid, sulfuric acid, quinine, iodine, chlorine, calcium, and even salt, all in different concentrations and several combinations. Eventually he settled on mercuric chloride, a powerful acid that had been avoided as a disinfectant because it was considered an outright poison. But his experiments showed that, when significantly diluted, with up to five thousand parts water, it killed microbes quickly and could then be safely rinsed away with water. Rather than take Koch's work as an affront, Lister was entirely grateful, and he soon altered his own methods accordingly.

Koch and his colleagues continued to push for disinfection, moving on from antisepsis (disinfecting a wound directly) to asepsis (sterilizing the surgical environment of implements and the operating environment). Soon, Koch's team had devised a process for steam sterilization that, even at short durations, completely killed any present bacteria. (As with other of Koch's breakthroughs, these procedures continue to be practiced today.)

In Paris, meanwhile, Pasteur kept pace. In 1880 he proved definitively that bacteria caused septicemia in the blood. In 1881, Koch published his new plating techniques, followed by Pasteur's work on infectious pleuropneumonia in cows and erysipelas in swine. In 1883, Koch's assistant Friedrich Loeffler identified the causal agent of diphtheria. And in 1885, Pasteur developed an effective vaccine for rabies. It was a remarkable time to be a bacteriologist, an era of apparently endless opportunity for discovery.

Though competition was an essential component of the Koch and Pasteur rivalry, internally each team thrived because of the closeness of the group. For his part, Pasteur recruited largely veterinarians and chemists, a preference that reflected his nonmedical background, while Koch recruited biologists and physicians for his lab. This gave each team a shared philosophy and likewise guided them in certain directions. Koch's group, steeped in *Wissenschaft*, excelled at the minutiae of the microscope, the exacting process of identification and confirmation. Pasteur's team was more focused on applications than technique. (Pasteur famously said that all science is applied science, a sentiment that would have been intuitive among his group but that would have seemed beside the point for Koch's team.) This steered the French team toward work that, in 1885, led to the vaccination for rabies, even though it would be decades before the causative agent (a virus, not a bacterium) was identified.

As the competition between Paris and Berlin increased, the

cooperation within the two teams must have been a ste▨
driving the team members to work harder and har▨
nights and families in order to push themselves to a ▨
Pasteur and Koch's would be one of the great rivalries of scien▨
and without the rivalry, there would have been far less science. The
two men may have been from competing schools and may have had
different dogmas, but they were fellow revolutionaries. Their every
discovery made it more difficult for other scientists to continue doubt-
ing the germ theory.

Of course, as with any revolution, there would be holdouts and
counterrevolutionaries. Into the 1880s and '90s, plenty of noteworthy
scientists denounced Koch and Pasteur equally as mischief-makers.
As late as 1883, Michel Peter, a Parisian physician held in high esteem
by his colleagues, went so far as to denounce Pasteur's work to his
face, at an address at the National Academy of Medicine. "What do I
care about your microbes? . . . I have said, and I repeat, that all this
research on microbes are not worth the time spent on them or the
fuss made about them, and that after all the work nothing would be
changed in medicine, there would only be a few extra microbes.
Medicine . . . is threatened by the invasion of incompetent, and rash
persons given to dreaming."

But as the discoveries mounted, these holdouts were increasingly
marginalized. Every discovery chipped away at the skepticism—and
created new expectations for science. Increasingly, there was a reason
to believe that science and medicine could explain things, that they
could create solutions to the ailments of humanity. Pasteur himself
boldly claimed, "It is within the power of man to eradicate infection
from the earth."

This, more than the individual discoveries of any one bacterium,
was the real revolution. Bacteriology was, in today's parlance, a platform for innovation, one that could apparently be used for various challenges and, with enough work and discipline, produce a result.

As the race between Koch and Pasteur took on greater stakes, och realized the rhetoric wasn't getting him anywhere; in fact, it was distracting him from the laboratory. What he needed was a new breakthrough. It wasn't enough to develop procedural innovations and mechanical improvements; it wasn't enough to publish significant but incremental discoveries. He needed something dramatic. He needed a discovery that could establish, definitively, his leadership in science—and, along the way, his primacy over Pasteur. He needed to move beyond the small stakes of a disease such as anthrax, which had a great economic cost in lost livestock but a human death toll of a few hundred annually, to one that deeply affected humanity, with a death toll in the millions.

What he needed, he realized, was a disease so ubiquitous, so pervasive, and so deadly that it was almost invisible.

CHAPTER 4

1882 · The Breakthrough

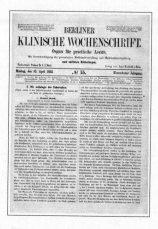

"The Etiology of Tuberculosis," Robert Koch's paper, published in 1882

On the brisk evening of March 24, 1882, Robert Koch left his rooms at the Imperial Health Office, walked across the Spree River, and headed toward the University of Berlin's Physiology Institute, a hulking caramel brick building a few blocks to the south. He was carrying boxes of equipment and specimens, but he couldn't tote the load by himself; his assistant Friedrich Loeffler shared the burden. As they walked, Koch volunteered that he was nervous. He was about to demonstrate an important discovery, a finding so startling that he scarcely expected anybody to believe him. At the least, he told Loeffler, he anticipated all sorts of quarreling to follow, "a year of hard battle."

Arriving at the institute, Koch and Loeffler climbed a few stairs to the library, where the demonstration would take place. The room was lined floor to ceiling with glass-doored bookshelves, each stocked with scientific journals, decades of estimable research that Koch was about to make obsolete, all at once. In the front of the room, Koch began laying his equipment out upon a large wooden table, an array of microscopes, test tubes, flasks, and tissue specimens taken from a variety of animals. Finally, he laid out dozens of small glass plates smeared with a white gelatin film, each containing a bacteria culture.

In the middle of the room, a large conference table held a dozen or so chairs, but as the room filled up, the table was moved to the side, until finally there were more than a hundred men standing elbow to elbow. The most eminent scientists in Germany were there. Some were admirers of Koch, who after less than two years in Berlin had established himself as a man to be watched. Paul Ehrlich was among these. Years earlier, he had witnessed Koch's anthrax demonstrations in Breslau, and he was now a junior member of Koch's team. Soon he would go on to develop the field of immunology; in 1908 he would win the Nobel Prize in medicine.

Others were skeptics; for them, Koch's germ theory was far from settled science. Chief among these was Rudolf Virchow, Berlin's "professor of professors," who stood, quiet and stern, among the others in the room. Years earlier, Koch had admired Virchow, even taking a special trip to Berlin during medical school to hear him lecture on physiology. But as a professional, Virchow had given Koch nothing but grief. As Koch's work grew more influential and as his stature in Berlin grew, Virchow had publicly scorned both, deeming the germ theory inessential for medicine. It was a mean insult, one that Koch couldn't help but take personally.

Few of the men there, whether friends or rivals, knew exactly what Koch would present that evening. Aside from his lecture's vague title, "On Tuberculosis," he had given up nothing in advance. But such was his reputation that every scientist in Berlin wanted to see what the wily Koch would come up with next.

With Koch's preparations complete, the doors were closed and the crowd settled down. Koch, clearly nervous, his spectacles perched

on his nose, shuffled his papers. "Die Tuberculose," he said, a
began to read his paper slowly, with frequent pauses, not for effe
as if to find his place. Later, Loeffler recalled the scene. "Koch wa
no means a dynamic lecturer who would overwhelm his audience
with brilliant words," he said. "He spoke slowly and haltingly, but
what he said was clear, simple, logically stated—in short, pure un-
adulterated gold."

Koch began by putting the disease in context, reminding his
audience of the vast toll that tuberculosis had taken on humanity. "If
the importance of a disease for mankind is measured by the number
of fatalities it causes," he said,

> then tuberculosis must be considered much more important
> than those most feared infectious diseases, plague, cholera,
> and the like. One in seven of all human beings dies from tu-
> berculosis. If one only considers the productive middle-age
> groups, tuberculosis carries away one third and often more of
> these.

Then he described his efforts to study the disease, how he had
tried to isolate and identify a specific cause. The first challenge was to
see the germ; in contrast to other bacteria he had worked with, Koch
had found this one elusive under his scope. The usual technique, developed by Paul Ehrlich, was to stain the slide of bacteria with a drop
of methylene blue dye. Typically, the cell walls of the bacteria absorb
some of the dye, and the rods and spores show up in relief on the
slide. But methylene blue didn't work here—until Koch ingeniously
added a *second*, brown dye. Suddenly, the bacteria were exposed, as if
a black light had been shone upon invisible ink.

Now that the bacteria were visible, he said, the experiments could
begin. He explained how he had cultured the bacteria and then injected them into a menagerie of healthy animals. These all developed
tuberculosis, one after the other, and he then began to isolate the

bacteria from their blood and tissue and inoculate them into more animals. When these, too, acquired the disease, he knew that he had isolated the true cause of tuberculosis.

Koch's presentation was labored, even tedious. He showed his test tubes and slides. He displayed his cultures. And he explained how he had tested and retested his work. He had anticipated every critique, every concern, and worked until he had the data to refute all arguments. His presentation that evening was a catalog of experimentation and self-examination, with Koch chalking up a finding only after he had presented the exhaustive evidence that would allow him to proceed. Throughout, his face remained stern and without emotion. There was no hand waving. There were no assumptions, no insinuations. There was only evidence and explanation—and finally, an end.

"All of these facts taken together can lead to only one conclusion," Koch said. "That the bacilli which are present in the tuberculosis substances not only accompany the tuberculosis process but are the cause of it. In the bacilli we have, therefore, the actual infective cause of tuberculosis."

The statement was so simply phrased, so matter-of-fact in its delivery, that the gravity of Koch's claim seemed almost benign. Here was Koch, who had gotten his start with jury-rigged equipment and kitchen-sink experiments, claiming to have discovered the cause of one of the most dire diseases in history. Here was Koch saying that this contagion was definitively a bacterium.

Nobody quite seemed to know what to make of this. There was no applause, no murmuring, no debate. The crowd was simply, utterly, absolutely speechless. Ehrlich was awestruck by the thoroughness and incontrovertibility of Koch's presentation. "I hold that evening to be the most important experience of my scientific life," he said later.

Some shook hands with Koch, offering him congratulations. Others moved to his materials, examining the cultures and slides under the scope. Then, finally, Virchow, the great paragon of German science, put on his hat and walked out of the room without saying a word.

To grasp the significance of Koch's discovery, we must first get our heads around this: To live in the nineteenth century was to experience infectious disease as a constant, to have unexplained illnesses afflict and dispatch loved ones without warning. Simply put, more people died of more things back then than do now; the death rate in London in 1850 was twenty-five per thousand—more than five times today's death rate.

Such an existence is, admittedly, almost inconceivable today. In the twenty-first century—in the developed world, at least—infectious disease is more a threat than a reality. In fact, we have been inoculated from the experience of contagion, the absolute routine drudgery of it, protected from the experience of a disease flourishing in our midst without any explanation, treatment, or cure. Today, few of us have much experience with infectious disease, beyond the occasional cold or flu or stomach bug.

When a contagion does cross our consciousness, it's either the stuff of distant Third World endemics such as malaria or, when in our midst, the stuff of front-page panics such as SARS. A sudden outbreak of disease—West Nile virus, say, or cholera or salmonella—appears to us like a breach in a force field, an aberration that we expect some authority will address and stamp out before it comes close to threatening us or our families. HIV/AIDS has killed about 620,000 Americans since the first case in 1981, roughly the same number of those who die from heart disease or cancer every year. This isn't to minimize the grave toll of HIV/AIDS. But by historical standards, the impact demonstrates how detached we are from the experience of infectious disease and how terrifying an epidemic can be today, even for those with little risk.

The nineteenth century, though, was a one-hundred-year dirge from one horrid epidemic to another. Six waves of cholera ravaged the globe during the century: The first killed hundreds of thousands from

e second killed 100,000 in France, 55,000 in the United
, and 150,000 in the United States; the third claimed 250,000
in Spain and nearly a million in Russia; and so on. There was
plague, too: In the 1850s, the "third pandemic" of bubonic fever broke
out in Asia, killing more than 12 million in China and India before
spreading worldwide. (It took nearly fifty years to reach North
America, breaking out in San Francisco's Chinatown district in 1900.)
And despite Jenner's vaccine, smallpox would periodically take advantage of vulnerable populations and kill off thousands before officials could mount an immunization response. Yellow fever, influenza,
measles—all these pulsed through growing urban populations of the
1800s, killing thousands and then stealthily retreating for a generation or two, waiting for immunity to fade, before returning to kill
thousands more. All these diseases came quickly, in terms of both
their attack on the human body and the speed with which they spread
through a community. They were fast and terrifying, and then, after
some weeks or months or at most a couple of years, they were gone.

Tuberculosis was altogether different. It was not an epidemic but
an *endemic* disease. It didn't come in waves or explode through a population; its presence was constant, pervasive, and persistent. Indeed,
the history of humanity is intertwined with the history of tuberculosis; it has been found in Egyptian mummies and in ancient Native
American burial grounds, and it is mentioned in four-thousand-year-
old Sanskrit texts from India. It likely emerged with the dawn of agriculture. Since the bacterium can survive in dust and dirt but dies
under sunlight, it seems probable that its origins lie in the soil itself.
(In this, it is not unlike anthrax.) From there, it was likely transmitted
to humans by the milk and meat of grazing livestock. (Cow's milk
was a vector for tuberculosis until pasteurization became widespread
in the early twentieth century.)

Though it had afflicted humanity for millennia, in the nineteenth
century tuberculosis went on a rampage, a tide of death known at the

time as the White Plague. As Koch noted in his opening remarks, the disease was the largest killer by far in the United States and Europe. At the Hôpital de la Charité in Paris, more than one-third of autopsies performed in the early 1800s found the cause of death to be TB. By the end of the century, in 1890, the registrar general of Ireland's returns showed that nearly half of those who died between fifteen and thirty-five years of age died of consumption. This toll was particularly painful for the nascent life insurance industry. In 1865, the British Empire Mutual Life calculated that tuberculosis was responsible for more than three-quarters of company benefit payments.

Year after year, the disease claimed a massive portion of the population, festering in families and neighborhoods and cities. It was always there, always taking lives in a steady attrition that made it seem, well, normal. To die of tuberculosis was, oftentimes, tantamount to just plain dying—it was how most people went. Charles Dickens, in 1839's *Nicholas Nickleby*, captures the despondency it brought on:

> There is a dread disease which so prepares its victim, as it were, for death; which so refines it of its grosser aspect, and throws around familiar looks unearthly indications of the coming change; a dread disease, in which the struggle between soul and body is so gradual, quiet, and solemn, and the result so sure, that day by day, and grain by grain, the mortal part wastes and withers away, so that the spirit grows light and sanguine with its lightening load, and, feeling immortality at hand, deems it but a new term of mortal life; a disease in which death and life are so strangely blended, that death takes the glow and hue of life, and life the gaunt and grisly form of death; a disease which medicine never cured, wealth never warded off, or poverty could boast exemption from; which sometimes moves in giant strides, and sometimes at a tardy sluggish pace, but, slow or quick, is ever sure and certain.

The tenacity of tuberculosis, the fact that it was "a disease which medicine never cured, wealth never warded off," made many physicians reluctant even to try. The English physician Thomas Young explained with resignation in 1815 that it was "a disease so frequent as to carry off prematurely about one-fourth part of the inhabitants of Europe, and so fatal as often to deter the practitioner even from attempting a cure." Writing in 1840, George Bodington, a physician who ran a sanatorium in Birmingham, England, bemoaned the general state of medical care for people with tuberculosis: "Consumptive patients are still lost as heretofore; they are considered hopeless and desperate cases by most practitioners, and the treatment commonly is conducted upon such an inefficient plan as scarcely to retard the fatal catastrophe." Bodington himself argued vociferously that a remote, dry climate, where the patient could be free of worry, offered some hope; his evangelism marked the beginning of the sanatorium movement in Europe and the United States.

All told, the pervasiveness of tuberculosis and the impotence of medicine to treat it created a specter of misery in nineteenth-century Europe and America. To live in this environment would have been always to be reminded of the presence of death. The constant cough of tuberculars, combined with the crackling sound of their lungs straining to breathe—a sound known as a rale—created a white noise of illness in European and American cities. The only consolation would have been ignorance: Until Koch's discovery of the bacillus, being coughed on, as many inevitably were, would not have prompted much concern.

The experience of the disease was, as Dickens described, typically a slow, dispiriting decline. Early symptoms were elusive; some cited "severe bodily or mental fatigue," while others described "a short and insidious cough, with a feeling of lassitude, and a decline in general health." Eventually a physician would confirm the diagnosis with his stethoscope but could offer little in the way of relief. A consumptive patient could live for years, even decades, with the disease, the cough coming and going in fits while, in the lungs, the bacteria slowly spread, eating away at the soft tissue. In its torpid pace, tuberculosis is more like the chronic diseases of today, such as heart disease or diabetes, which can take years to whittle away at the body before dealing a fatal blow.

In the closing years of the nineteenth century, tuberculosis was at its most rapacious. One can get a sense of how ubiquitous it was by noting how many famous figures of the day died from it. Elizabeth Barrett Browning, Johann Wolfgang von Goethe, Friedrich Schiller, Henry David Thoreau, all three Brontë sisters, Anton Chekhov, Washington Irving, Guy de Maupassant, Edgar Allan Poe, Sir Walter Scott . . . The toll is so vast that there's an entire Wikipedia entry devoted to the subject.

Such rolls of notables convinced many that consumption had its upside. The slow, wasting nature of the disease made it fodder for romanticists and drove the plots of operas such as *La Traviata* and *La Bohème*. It infused the poetry of Keats, Shelley, and Byron. "I look pale," Byron told a guest in Patras in 1828. "I should like to die of consumption." "Why?" his guest asked. "Because the ladies would all say, 'Look at that poor Byron, how interesting he looks in dying!'"

The truth was far less beautiful and far more brutal. Nineteenth-century civilization seems to have been custom-designed for a microbe such as tuberculosis. It was, of course, the great age of industrialization, when people were pouring into European and American cities for work. To say they lived on top of one another is to be fairly literal: The average household size in 1850s England was nearly seven persons, more than double the average today.

Inside these "fever-breeding structures," as journalist and social reformer Jacob Riis described them, the levels of cleanliness were, by today's standards, abysmal: Lice and bedbugs were common. Working people typically wore the same clothes for days, and for many families, soap was still a novelty. (In the United Kingdom, use of soap was about three and a half pounds per person annually in 1801 but would grow to five times that amount, nearly fifteen pounds per person, by century's end.) With no plumbing, water was drawn and carried from local pumps and so was scarce.

Outside, on the streets, the gutters were full of household waste and the piss and shit of animals, from humans to horses. Even in cities that did have some sewers, such as Paris, sanitation was horrendous. During the "Great Stink" in 1880, the sewer under the boulevard de Rochechouart clogged up with human excrement. The fumes were so concentrated that four men sent underground to clear the stuff died of asphyxiation. (London had its own Great Stink, in 1858, when the Thames overflowed with sewage.)

And then there was the spit. Spitting in the nineteenth century was as routine as chewing gum is today. Clearing one's throat and hawking the mucus onto the street was not just common; it was considered by many to be outright proper. Swallowing one's expectorant, on the contrary, was considered unhealthy. "Why do we expectorate?" asked an editorial in *The Medical Brief*, an American journal. "Because the passages are filled with dead matter which the system seeks to eliminate. Nature knows no laws but her own. She directs the individual expectorate, while the profession who has charge of his physical welfare wants to force him to transfer this dead matter to the stomach to deprave the gastric juice, and further harm the system."

Americans, perhaps not surprisingly, were considered the worst offenders, what with their appetite for tobacco and their generally uncouth culture. Alfred Bunn, an English writer visiting the United States in 1853, observed spitting, well, everywhere:

> They spit, as a matter of course, upon floors, and even costly carpets covering them; in grates, over, or under them; in all public conveyances, all about the streets, in shops, on the decks and in the cabins of all vessels, in theatres and other places of amusement, in both Houses of Congress, all lobbies leading thereto, and all apartments connected therewith; at

all tables, during all meals, in their counting-houses and stores, in passages and bedrooms, which makes it an impossibility to cross them, without either putting on slippers, or "putting your foot in it"; and as no place is sacred from pollution, of course they spit in their Courts of Justice, there being no law against it.

In truth, spitting was routine throughout the United States *and* Europe. Part of this was not just social but simply environmental, a consequence of cities, such as London, being covered with a pall of dust and smoke. An 1847 French medical textbook reported that "many persons, in health, every morning reject several sputa, of a grayish or blackish color; this color is owing to the smoke which collects from lamps, candles, etc., particularly in small apartments." Indeed, the amount of spit hawked up in London every day was used as an argument *against* the germ theory in the months after Koch's discovery. "When we consider the number of consumptive people who, being under no restriction, go about coughing and expectorating freely in the streets and parks of London," wrote C. J. B. Williams of Brompton Hospital in the *British Medical Journal*, "we must admit that the bacilli, though ever present, are not very active in ill-doing."

Alas, Dr. Williams couldn't have been more wrong. All this hawking and expectorating was, in fact, exceptionally kind to the tuberculosis microbe. When a diseased person spits (or coughs or sneezes or even talks), a cloud of saliva droplets fills the air. In each droplet are thousands of bacteria, coming along for the ride. Even when a neighbor inhales this emission, the odds of the bacteria causing infection are fairly low. The relative bulk of the cloud of droplets means that most get stuck in nasal mucus or the higher respiratory tract, never making their way to the soft spot of the lungs. But some of these droplets linger in the air, and the air evaporates the saliva. The residue, known as droplet nuclei, can continue to float in the air, ready to be drawn by some newcomer's inhalation, and are small enough to be sucked deeply into the lungs.

Even then, the victim isn't yet doomed. The lungs are filled with special immune cells primed to absorb invasive bacteria and destroy them. Tuberculosis, though, is well equipped for this battle. The bacterium has a notably thick, waxy cell wall, which makes it difficult for white blood cells to penetrate and destroy the invader. Instead, the body takes a secondary defense measure: It surrounds the bacteria and locks them into nodules, known as granulomas, a kind of stalemate between bacteria and host. For 90 percent of those exposed to tuberculosis, this is as far as the bacteria will get. These cases are considered latent tuberculosis, as the disease is present but inactive; most persons will never know they harbor the germ.

But for the unlucky 10 percent, the bacterium breaks down the granuloma, outstripping the body's defenses, and begins to reproduce and spread. In classic consumption, the bacteria fester slowly, consuming the thin, soft tissue of the air sacs in the lungs. If the germs migrate and attack a blood vessel, this creates the "damned spot" John Keats saw one day on his handkerchief. ("It is arterial blood," he wrote a friend a year before his death from consumption. "That drop of blood is my death warrant. I must die.") But if the rot stays in the tissue, the bacteria continue their march through the body, month after month, year after year. Besides the telltale cough, sometimes the bacteria spread to the surface of the body, creating sores and abscesses on the skin; sometimes they moved to other internal organs, causing inflammation and threatening organ function. In some nineteenth-century victims, the bacteria ate away at bone, a particularly painful development. (A dreadful, and typical, treatment in the nineteenth century was to open the bone to the air, with the hope that the pus would drain and, somehow, the patient would heal. It didn't work.) And all along, one patient would spread it to another, and to another, keeping the disease alive even as the victims died.

Today's epidemiologists have a metric for quantifying the contagiousness of a disease, known as the basic reproduction number. Denoted as R_0, it designates how many people one contagious individual is likely to transmit disease to during the course of his illness. If the R_0 falls below 1, then the disease will die out on its own; if the R_0 is above 1, it will continue to spread through a population. The higher the R_0, the faster a disease spreads and the harder it is to control. A disease such as influenza actually has a fairly low R_0, around 2, while the R_0 of HIV is between 2 and 5. Measles and pertussis, meanwhile, can be extremely contagious, each with an R_0 over 15 commonly. (This is one reason public health officials are so adamant about vaccinating against these diseases: They must be kept out of a population altogether, since once they take hold, they're extremely difficult to extinguish.) In the late nineteenth century, tuberculosis had an R_0 of somewhere around 3, making it a tenacious if not explosive disease. That is comparable with viruses such as smallpox and polio, tuberculosis's most common cousins, historically speaking. But the R_0 is calculated over the *lifetime* of the illness for the diseased individual. Since smallpox and polio make quick work of their victims, these ancillary infections happen in a relatively brief time span. Tuberculosis, though, is a long-festering disease, twice over: People can live their whole lives with it in a latent, or dormant, state, and they can live with the disease in an active state for many years, if not decades. The R_0 value for tuberculosis, then, reflects the disease's constancy and tenacity.

In the nineteenth century, in typical urban conditions, tuberculosis bacteria would be just about everywhere. They would be on food, on walls, on forks and plates and spoons. They would be on the communal drinking cups fastened on public water pumps. They would be, practically speaking, unavoidable. Given the high mortality rate for TB—66 percent of active cases would end in death—the math says that practically everyone in the nineteenth century carried the bacteria in his or her body. Who might go on to develop the disease— well, that was a trickier matter.

This was the error of Dr. Williams and so many others who argued against the contagiousness of tuberculosis. Williams thought he had evidence on his side: His Brompton Hospital for Consumption, in London, had specialized in the care and treatment of consumptives since the 1840s, and the hospital had closely tracked its cases, from symptoms to outcomes. According to these data, there seemed to be little signs of *contagion* in TB cases, in the sense of being able to track the disease from one individual to another. Indeed, the hospital staff themselves were in generally good health and had relatively fewer cases of TB than the public, Williams estimated. If the disease were contagious, surely that wouldn't be the case.

But what Williams and his Brompton colleagues couldn't see— what they didn't know they could look for (the microbe)—was still there, quietly doing its work. Dr. Williams assumed that infections happened quickly, as in a measles outbreak. But tuberculosis works more slowly and stealthily. Indeed, it was the *casualness* of consumption—the fact that husbands could have it when their wives seemingly did not, for instance—that baffled those considering the matter.

This almost aloof pace of consumption made it exceedingly difficult for medical men to perceive it as a contagion akin to diseases such as smallpox and whooping cough. In an 1864 paper entitled "Is Consumption Ever Contagious?" Dr. Henry Bowditch, a Boston physician, noted the slow development of cases he had treated. "If contagion had anything really to do with it," he observed, "why did it prove so long in showing itself? Usually contagion shows itself soon. This was months in developing itself." Bowditch's conclusion adroitly skirts the question he posed; he decided that "consumption is not *contagious* in the usual acceptation of that word," but, he added, "it might be *infectious*." Using the alternate term *phthisis*, he concluded his paper with a description of the disease that could pass, today, as a fair expression of the basic reproductive number for tuberculosis. "By long attendance of the closest kind, by inhaling the breath of the phthisical patient, by living in the phthisical atmosphere, so to speak, and in general by a neglect of hygienic laws during such attendance, the health may be undermined and phthisis set in." But whether this was the work of a germ—well, that was too speculative even to consider.

Koch's discovery was the definitive answer to Bowditch's question, the solution to a mystery that had long dogged science. But it was a mystery that many would have denied even existed; after all, medicine already had perfectly reasonable explanations for consumption. Koch's explanation was, for skeptics, just one more thrown onto the pile. "There is hardly any pathological question that has been so swayed by every wind of doctrine as this of tubercle," lamented Dr. Sidney Coupland in an address to the Middlesex Hospital two months before Koch announced his discovery. "Not even the subject of inflammation has been viewed from so many standpoints, and received so many and varied explanations."

This disease, which the seventeenth-century writer John Bunyan called "the captain of all the men of death," was thought, at various times, to stem from bad climate and from sloth. Most of all, it was considered hereditary, brought on by one's family background. The hereditary theory for TB dated back to Hippocrates, who noted that "consumptives beget consumptives." It would prove an exceptionally hard notion to shake, insofar as the disease *did* spread through families, with the onset between family members often occurring generationally, delayed by years or decades. What's more, the symptoms of consumption (lassitude, lack of appetite, emaciation) seemed to endorse the notion that a consumptive had inherited an overall physical weakness that culminated in the disease, rather than the other way around.

There was something to this notion. Recall that everyone in major cities was surely exposed to the bacterium, but only a fraction of those would develop the disease. Those who did were the weaker and more vulnerable, their immune systems less able to fight off the contagion.

In that way, one's inherited traits *were* an obvious factor in the disease. When the next generation started to show similar signs of weakness, it seemed obvious that the parents' tendency toward poor health had simply been passed on to their spawn.

The hereditary theory found an inadvertent ally in Charles Darwin, who began publishing his notions of inheritance in the 1830s. Darwin's ideas about natural selection and the survival of the fittest appeared to neatly explain why consumption might run in some families and not others. An 1872 essay by Dr. James Ross of Manchester, elaborately titled *The Graft Theory of Disease, Being an Application of Mr. Darwin's Hypothesis of Pangenesis to the Explanation of the Phenomena of the Zymotic Diseases* ("zymotic" referred to acute diseases, such as TB, that seemed to spread), overtly rejected speculation that some contagion caused tuberculosis. Dr. Ross, a prolific author of wrongheaded medical treatises, found in Darwin's theories a much more satisfying explanation:

> In developing certain qualities by sexual selection, man has also produced a tendency to disease and more especially to tubercular disease. . . . In the prosecution of this design, Mr. Darwin's hypothesis of Pangenesis, by means of which he explains the various forms of genesis, inheritance reversion, and the phenomena of budding and grafting, was adopted because an hypothesis by which these great operations carried out through the whole biological series can be explained is much more deserving of credit than one specially constructed for the explanation of a more limited set of phenomena.

The fact that Darwin's work—just a few decades previous considered a heresy not just to science, but also to religion and all things sacred—was now being deployed as an argument against the emerging heresy of microbes was, to say the least, ironic. (Darwin himself died just three weeks after Koch's discovery of the tuberculosis bacterium and therefore never addressed the debate.)

As was the case with Darwin's work when it was misapplied, the hereditary explanation for tuberculosis compounded the stigma of the disease. If tuberculosis was a manifestation of weakness, of poor stock, then consumptives were clearly genetically inferior creatures. In regard to patients with scrofula, the manifestation of tuberculosis on the skin, Dr. Ross put the argument plainly: "On an average, those who have the scrofulous diathesis are deficient in the intellectual and active mental characteristics, which give to their possessor a calm judgment, indomitable courage, and perseverance—the qualities which will ensure success in an open struggle for existence against all competitors." The fact that cases of tuberculosis had been *increasing* during his century (that pesky R_o again), rather than being selected against and thus decreasing, didn't seem to register with Dr. Ross. It seemed that he and others somehow hoped that consumptives might just go away on their own. It was a heavy burden to place on fully one-quarter of the population.

Among those who believed in the hereditary origins of tuberculosis was Rudolf Virchow, who considered the disease to be a form of cancer, the tubercles in the lungs appearing to him as a sort of tumor. *All disease from cells,* Virchow believed, a mantra that consumption seemed to obey, given the tendency of the disease to migrate throughout the body—it seemed analogous to how cancer malignancies spread from organ to organ. Virchow's argument packed considerable weight in medicine, and his explanation was routinely cited as definitive.

The similarity with cancer made sense, in part, because tuberculosis had radically different manifestations in different regions of the body. Just as the taxonomy of cancer is still today governed by its area of affliction (colon cancer, pancreatic cancer, breast cancer, and so on), so TB then had been carved into several different diseases, depending on where it occured. The most common form was pulmonary tuberculosis, where it was known as consumption, or phthisis. When it turned up in the lymph system, revealing itself through swollen glands in the neck and eventually forming ulcers on the skin, it was called scrofula. This form of TB most commonly developed from drinking raw milk, which, in the days before pasteurization, could contain bovine tuberculosis, a closely related form of the disease in cattle. On the skin, it was known as lupus (or, more formally, *Lupus vulgaris,* in contrast to the autoimmune condition known today as *Lupus erythematosus*). In each incarnation of TB, it was possible to locate tubercles (waxy sacs of bacteria and pus that resembled a particularly odious cheese), but there was great debate whether these diseases were related or distinct phenomena. Add up the victims of all of them, though, and tuberculosis is believed to be the most lethal disease in history, having claimed more than a billion lives since it was first identified in ancient Greece.

Virchow, the greatest pathologist and surgeon of his day—he was also a pioneering hygienist, having led the charge to clean up the water supply in Berlin and other German cities—was acting according to the best principles of pathology. His understanding of disease was rooted in direct empirical observation: He looked under his microscope and saw distinct growths. And when he looked at these signs and symptoms, he saw clear distinctions and differences among the various conditions. All this was similar to how cancer worked in the body, and since cancer was a known disease, surely it made more sense to attribute the growths to a known disease than to make up some other mechanism.

Koch's discovery, though, proved that despite outward resemblances between cancer and tuberculosis, the internal mechanisms were entirely different. What's more, all tubercles, whether in consumption or scrofula or lupus, contained *Mycobacterium tuberculosis*—one disease caused by one pathogen. In a single presentation, built on just a few months of lab work, Koch had rendered obsolete libraries of medical textbooks representing decades of work by thousands of men.

It was the first time that a pathological understanding of disease—the one that Virchow had spent his career establishing—was surpassed by a biological one.

Koch's *Mycobacterium tuberculosis* didn't solve just one mystery—what causes tuberculosis?—but many mysteries at once. He had found a tiny, elusive microbe just two or three microns long (the period at the end of this sentence is about six hundred microns long). Yet the size of the microbe was in inverse proportion to the magnitude of his discovery. The latter was so big, so transcendentally significant, that hereafter it couldn't be avoided in medicine.

But it must be acknowledged: Koch wasn't, in fact, the first. More than 150 years before, the English physician Benjamin Marten had suggested that some sort of minuscule animal might be the cause of the disease. Marten had observed too many coincidences, where one consumptive's passing acquaintance with others had left them with the affliction. That relationship couldn't be explained, he felt, except by something exchanged between the people involved—and this, he surmised, might certainly be a creature: "If the Blood and Juices of such distemper'd People, be charg'd with vast quantities of Animalcula, as I have conjectur'd, then their profuse sweats, and their Breath also, may be likewise charg'd with them, or their Ova or Eggs, which by that means may possibly be covey'd into the Bodies of those who lie, or are most conversant with them." Though Marten had committed his proposal to print, his argument held no sway with his contemporaries.

Nor did the enterprising epidemiology of William Budd carry much weight when he made a keen analysis of tuberculosis cases in Africa in 1867. Budd, who practiced medicine in the shipping port of Bristol, England, had noticed that a steady stream of African patients developed tuberculosis while working on British ships. After a series of investigations, he realized that this was widespread. "Everywhere along the African sea-board, where the blacks have come into contact and intimate relations with the whites, phthisis causes a large mortality among them." But he had learned from none other than Dr. Livingstone (of "Stanley and Livingstone" fame) that in the interior of the continent, "where intercourse with Europeans has been limited to casual contact . . . there is reason to believe that phthisis does not exist." Budd surmised that Europeans must be the vector for the disease, an astute act of epidemiology, if not politics. The disease, he argued in *The Lancet,* "is disseminated through specific germs contained in the tuberculous matter cast off by persons already suffering from the disease." Budd's observations, though well-founded, were apparently too divorced from the experience of most doctors to yield any practical result.

The most substantial predecessor had been Jean-Antoine Villemin, a French army surgeon who, in the 1860s, conducted a series of experiments testing whether tuberculosis could be transmitted from one animal to another. Villemin's interest began when he observed how tuberculosis seemed to affect young men who moved to the city, even though they were previously healthy in their rural homes. He compared the effect to how glanders, a horse disease, seemed to spread when a team was yoked together. "The phthisical soldier is to his messmates what the glandered horse is to its yoke fellow," Villemin conjectured.

He soon went beyond conjecture. In an experiment, he injected healthy rabbits with fluid from the lungs of a man who had died of TB. After three months, he killed the rabbits and examined their lungs. They were filled with tubercles. He conducted another experiment, this time taking tissue from a diseased cow and injecting it into rabbits. They got sick even faster. (This was the first experiment, as it happens, to explore the difference between the human and bovine forms of TB.) Villemin continued to run experiments, and in 1868 he published *Studies on Tuberculosis*, where he laid out evidence for his theory that tuberculosis could be spread from one animal to another.

He was exuberant about the implications of his research and began lobbying for a number of social reforms, including improved living and working conditions and thorough disinfection measures. "These are the ideas which should direct us in the research for curative and prophylactic measures in turberculosis," he wrote. "These are the hopes which our discovery luringly had held out for us."

But Villemin would be greatly disappointed. His work, while it did prompt some discussion, did not generate any fundamental changes. As later experiments by others failed to reproduce his results (almost certainly a result of their methods, not Villemin's), his work was increasingly considered dubious. In 1881, on the eve of Koch's presentation, Austin Flint issued the fifth edition of his textbook *The Principles and Practice of Medicine*. In its discussion of tuberculosis, the book dismissed any theories of contagion. "The doctrine of the contagiousness of the disease has . . . its advocates, but general belief is in its non-communicability." And then came Koch, whose evidence, assembled over many months in the laboratory in Berlin, was enough to shift the burden of proof the other way.

Why did Koch's discovery resonate when his predecessors' theories had not? As Francis Darwin, Charles's son, observed, "In science the credit goes to the man who convinces the world, not to the man to whom the idea first occurs." In the face of profound disbelief, Villemin's science, as promising as it was, could not convince the world.

It's worth noting that Koch's paper does acknowledge Villemin's work in its very first words: "The discovery of Villemin that tuberculosis can be transmitted to animals has been confirmed a number of times." No sooner did he acknowledge the discovery, though, than he observed that it had proven unconvincing: "but has also been opposed on seemingly good grounds, so that up until recently it has not been possible to state for certain whether tuberculosis is an infectious disease or not."

Given credit or not, until his death in 1892, Villemin would hold a grudge. In 1882 he confessed to Pasteur that he felt Koch's glory had come at his own expense. "I have been so much discussed, so often attacked, that I suffer a certain amount of distress in thinking that the leading scientific academy still gives, at least, a sort of toleration to my former enemies. . . . Koch will enter the Académie des Sciences through widely flung doors, in the triumphant way that has made a conquest of him of all the honours of his country."

Villemin might as well have been fighting the movement of the spheres. His complaint—that Koch, who had gotten so much glory, was getting still more—is known today as the Matthew effect. The term was coined by Robert Merton in a 1968 paper in *Science*: "The Matthew effect consists in the accruing of greater increments of recognition for particular scientific contributions to scientists of considerable repute and the withholding of such recognition from scientists who have not yet made their mark." (The term gets its name from a passage in the Gospel of Matthew: "For unto every one that hath shall be given, and he shall have abundance: but from him that hath not shall be taken away even that which he hath.")

Villemin was partly right, insofar as Koch's research was quickly hailed around the world partially because Koch had established himself as a man of meticulous methods. But this is tautological in the sense that Koch's work on tuberculosis was *characteristically* meticulous. Yes, it helped that in the twenty years since Villemin's work, the germ theory had become much less speculative, with a growing weight of evidence behind it. But Koch, as much as anybody, had been responsible for creating that evidence. His postulates, which by now were well-established protocols in his laboratory work, were surely part of the winning argument. The links in the chain of evidence fit together.

ROBERT KOCH MAY HAVE EXPECTED A YEAR OF FIGHTING, BUT IT would not take a year to convince the world. His theory was, all at once, accepted as proven. Rarely had medicine ever experienced, wrote the *British Medical Journal*, "so sudden and complete casting aside of tradition." In a report published just a month after the Berlin demonstration, *The London Medical Gazette* cautiously praised Koch's work. "To those old-standing questions which have hitherto baffled the penetration of the wisest of our profession, Dr. Koch has returned an answer that is singularly free from ambiguity. Tuberculosis . . . is a parasitic disease of the internal organs; the parasite is a bacillus." (The *Gazette* editors were particularly pleased that Koch's work might create less tolerance for public spitting.)

Word of Koch's breakthrough took longer to cross the Atlantic, though, and by the time *The New York Times* caught wind of the discovery, in early May, the paper's correspondent was appropriately peeved that such essential news was just then reaching the States. "The rapid growth of the Continental capitals, the movements of princely noodles and fat, vulgar Duchesses, the debates in the Servian Skupschina, and the progress or receding of sundry royal gouts are given to the wings of the lightning; a lumbering mail-coach is swift enough for the news of one of the great scientific discoveries of the age." The paper went on to compare Koch to Darwin, praising him for giving "new force and meaning [to] the command, 'Know thyself.'"

But the *Times* dispatch also made clear that this was just the start of what it expected from Dr. Koch. The real glory would come with a treatment or a cure. "The popular interest in the little parasite Dr. Koch has introduced to the world will deepen in proportion as medical science demonstrates its power to annihilate him or rob him of his fatal power," suggesting inoculation as the most probable course.

This was indeed the new standard emerging for the germ hunters: not just discovery, but some sort of treatment or inoculation that might turn bacteriology from the academic to the pragmatic. Koch recognized this; now in the prime of his investigative powers and at the height of his self-regard—it was after his TB discovery, not surprisingly, that Koch uncorked his full fury against Pasteur—he was convinced that tuberculosis was the most likely candidate for such a cure. With his postulates, his analytic skills, and his technical prowess, he had the method down cold. Surely taking the next step, from pinpointing a cause to devising a remedy, was simply a matter of course. Pasteur had done it with anthrax, after all, and with inferior skills, resources, and procedures.

In the months following his discovery of *Mycobacterium tuberculosis*, Koch would be promoted by the kaiser and given a larger staff, a larger salary, and larger facilities. He would join the front ranks of scientists in Germany and Europe. And as he told his daughter, Gertrud, now thirteen years old and in boarding school, he would serve as the central attraction during the German Exposition of Hygiene and Public Health. "I have even had the privilege," he wrote, "of explaining bacteria to the Crown Prince, the Grand Duke of Baden, the King and Queen of Saxony, and many other royal personages." But he now had the thirst, and the confidence, to make another discovery, better than the last. Koch was determined: Tuberculosis was all his, and it would be he, not Pasteur, who captured the greater glory.

PART II

CHAPTER 5

1882 · The Doctor in Southsea

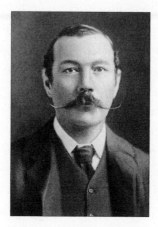

Arthur Conan Doyle, circa 1890

In June 1882, in the town of Southsea, a suburb of Portsmouth on the southern coast of England, Arthur Conan Doyle, just twenty-three years old, admired the bright brass plate newly affixed to his door. "Dr. Conan Doyle," it read. "Physician and Surgeon."

Conan Doyle smiled and then walked down the road to Southsea's high street, stopping in at the local newspaper. For a few pence, he placed a brief announcement in the next edition: "Dr. Doyle begs to notify that he has removed to 1 Bush Villas, Elm Grove, next to the Bush Hotel." Back home, he went to his front window and placed a red lamp, the traditional beacon of the British physician, on the sill. He struck a match and lit the lamp. Dr. Arthur Conan Doyle was ready for business.

Conan Doyle wasn't from the area; he had earned his medical

credentials in his hometown of Edinburgh, Scotland. Nonetheless, after earlier attempts to start a practice in Birmingham and Plymouth failed, he had fixed on greater Portsmouth as a possible perch and found Southsea, a growing seaside resort with pleasure piers, several hotels, and about thirty-four thousand residents. It looked like a promising spot, but there were already several doctors in town. So Conan Doyle began to chart a course. He bought a shilling map of the town, laid it out on a table in his hotel, and planned a series of walks. Day after day, he would amble up and down the roads of Southsea, trying never to pass along the same block twice. As he walked, he kept his eyes peeled for the brass plates and red lamps of the other doctors in Southsea: the competition. Soon he had covered every street in town.

"On my map I put a cross for every doctor," he would describe later. "So at the end of that time I had a complete chart of the whole place, and could see at a glance where there was a possible opening." That spot was 1 Bush Villas, tucked snuggly between the Bush Hotel and St. Paul's Baptist Church, and less than a mile from the Eye and Ear Hospital. Conan Doyle's technique was typically resourceful, if not a little ingenious. It wholly suited the man who would later create Sherlock Holmes, a character with those same attributes in spades.

Born in Edinburgh in 1859, of genteel middle-class Irish stock, Conan Doyle was the son of an alcoholic artist and the nephew of successful Irish scholars. (His uncle Henry would serve as director of the National Gallery of Ireland, in Dublin.) These uncles, both faithful Catholics and family men, had generously sponsored a robust Jesuit education for young Arthur, allowing him to go to school in Lancashire and Austria. Though he bristled at the religion, he took to the schooling; it fostered in him expectations typical of Britain's growing upper middle class.

In 1876 young Conan Doyle entered the University of Edinburgh's medical school, then as now considered one of the finest medical colleges in Europe. He went into medicine dutifully, if not passionately. It seemed a reasonable way to make good on the investments his family had placed in him and a way to avoid the wanton path his father had followed. When he graduated from medical school in 1881, Conan Doyle was a young man of honor, family responsibility, and most of all ambition. He seethed with the need to do *something* of distinction. But as it was for so many young men pining to make their mark, the world didn't yet know who he was and was rudely indifferent to his potential anyway. Instead of the glorious adventures he believed he was capable of, here he was trawling for business in Southsea, where every patient and every shilling were a struggle.

Physically, he was a big man—more than six feet tall and nearly two hundred pounds, with a sixteen-inch neck and a broad build befitting an occasional boxer—and wore a full mustache. While in medical school, he had taken leave to sign up as a ship's surgeon on a whaling expedition to the Arctic. It was the first great adventure of his life, and he had relished the physical challenge, learning how to harpoon whales and smash the skulls of seals. He had spent six months doctoring the crew, though his happiest moments were passed thrashing about with his shipmates. "I went on board the whaler a big, straggling youth, I came off it a powerful, well-grown man," he wrote in his memoirs.

So, after graduating school, he signed up for another tour as a ship's surgeon, this time aboard the steamship *Mayumba*, en route from Liverpool to West Africa. This was a far less satisfying journey, marred by fires aboard the ship and a bout of malaria. He returned to England after three months, grateful to have made it back alive.

Those adventures were long behind him by the time he'd gotten to Southsea. To pass the time, or to forget his loneliness, Conan Doyle would pick up his pen and write a story. It was a chance to drift away from his reality. His early stories mimicked his favorite boyhood authors, Sir Walter Scott and Edgar Allan Poe. His first story had been published in 1879, while he was still a medical student. "The Mystery of Sasassa Valley" involved a treasure hunt in South Africa (where he had yet to travel). In 1881 "A Night Among the Nihilists" took readers to Odessa (again, where Conan Doyle had never been) for a night with Russian millionaires. He wrote adventure tales of ghost ships and the jungles of Africa. Every once in a while, after many submissions, a story would even be published.

While his stories were full of imaginative details, his letters home were, on the contrary, strikingly pedestrian. To his mother, he would confess all the anxieties and concerns of a newly independent bachelor, providing a dutiful accounting of bills owed him and debts he owed others, and a nod to the occasional patient who rang his bell. "Just a line to say that we have had another lucky hit," he wrote to his mother in February 1883, just seven months into his Southsea practice. "A man broke his jaw & fractured his skull just outside the house today in a carriage accident . . . and I had to take him home and received 2 guineas for my trouble." If his stories contained Conan Doyle's dreams of where he aspired to be, his letters home were frank confessions of where he was.

In between were the letters he wrote to *The Lancet* and the *British Medical Journal*. In these, Conan Doyle drew on his meager caseload and his experiences in Edinburgh to offer (what he hoped would be) a novel scientific observation. While still in school, he'd had one such letter published, in the *BMJ*, chronicling his experiment (upon himself) in taking ever greater doses of *Gelsemium*, an herbal medicine related to strychnine. "I determined to ascertain how far one might go in taking the drug, and what the primary symptoms of an overdose might be." Conan Doyle boosted his dose steadily until, after a week, a severe depression and "diarrhoea . . . so persistent and prostrating" forced him to give up the experiment.

He'd had another bit of luck on March 25, 1882—the day after Koch's TB presentation, as it happened, though Conan Doyle would not have known this—when *The Lancet* published a case note on leucocythemia (an old term for leukemia). Technically, it was a letter to the editor, not a work of research, and to the chagrin of the exuberant young doctor, they got his name wrong, mistakenly crediting "A.

Cowan Doyle." Nonetheless, the letter was testimony to the fact that, though this physician had been living a circumscribed existence, he had his eyes on broader horizons.

In the days after Conan Doyle's letter was published, the British medical journals began to report on Koch's discovery of the tubercle bacterium. "The pathological importance of the discovery of the proximate cause of this frightful scourge of the human race cannot be over-estimated," *The Lancet* pronounced on April 22, 1882, "nor is it possible to foretell the practical results to which it may lead." For the rest of the year, scarcely a week passed without either *The Lancet* or the *BMJ* posting an update on Koch's work; in its retrospective issue for 1882, the *BMJ* hailed "the splendid series of researches by Koch" as "first in importance among the pathological work of the year."

Though the British journals seemed cautious about the broader implications of the germ theory (the *BMJ* rather more enthusiastic about the promise of bacteriological medicine than the conservative *Lancet*), both publications diligently covered what was undeniably a powerful idea with a growing body of compelling evidence behind it. If nothing else, clearly the news had shaken up the medical establishment. Both journals dutifully printed letters from august English physicians defending the long-standing theories that Koch's novel work would undercut. (Most were hesitant to give up their faith in the hereditary origins of tuberculosis, which seemed so self-evident in their clinical observations.) Others, such as Lister, looked at Koch's work and saw vindication. But the academic debate seemed increasingly petty compared to the pragmatic argument that, with this great killer of humanity finally identified, some progress might be made toward combating it.

Throughout the summer of 1882, "Koch's bacilli," as it began to be called, went on something of a road show in England, with microscopic exhibitions of the tuberculosis bacterium in Norwich, London, and other English cities. One such display, in June at the Royal College of Physicians in London, drew the attendance of two of

Queen Victoria's sons, the Duke of Albany and the Prince of Wales, who peered in the microscope to observe the bacteria and, it was reported, were duly impressed.

All this sparked something in Conan Doyle's imagination. He recognized that a new era was emerging, one where men were beginning to gain sight, and insight, into disease. So sometime in late 1882, he picked up his pen and began to write an essay conjuring a fanciful world where men were themselves microbes, set loose in the body:

> Had a man the power of reducing himself to the size of less than the one-thousandth part of an inch, and should he, while of this microscopic stature, convey himself through the coats of a living artery, how strange the sight that would meet his eye! All round him he would see a rapidly flowing stream of clear transparent fluid, in which many solid and well-defined bodies were being whirled along. . . . Here and there, however, on the outskirts of the throng, our infinitesimal spectator would perceive bodies of a very different character.

These are the opening words to "Life and Death in the Blood," an essay published in the popular journal *Good Words* in March 1883. The essay, essentially, was Conan Doyle's go at translating what he'd been reading in the medical journals for a literate but unscientific audience.

Conan Doyle found his material in the most exciting arena in medical science: the rivalry between Louis Pasteur and Robert Koch and their work identifying those things called germs. "The existence of these little organisms . . . may have been suspected by our forefathers," he wrote, assuming an authority on the page that he perhaps lacked in his practice. "But it is only in the last few years that their presence has been clearly demonstrated, and their relation to disease duly appreciated." Despite the Koch-Pasteur rivalry, he astutely noted, the two men were joined in the same goal, observing that "one great thinker stimulates the latent powers of many others." Though he was a world away from the great labs of Europe, Conan Doyle, writing from his lonely house, had put his finger on a major shift in medical science.

In a burst of imagination, the essay ended with a vision for the future of bacteriology. Noting Koch's insights into tuberculosis and Pasteur's vaccine for anthrax, Conan Doyle issued a bold challenge:

> Given that a single disease, proved to depend upon a parasitic organism, can be effectually and certainly stamped out, why should not all diseases depending upon similar causes be also done away with? That is the great question which the scientific world is striving to solve; and in the face of it how paltry do war and statecraft appear, and everything which fascinates the attention of the multitude! Let things go as they are going, and it is probable that in the days of our children's children, or even earlier, consumption, typhus, typhoid, cholera, malaria, scarlatina, diphtheria, measles, and a host of other diseases will have ceased to exist.

The essay was well received, helping the British public understand the purpose and potential impact of the European science.

THE LABORATORY IS A LONG WAY FROM THE DOCTOR'S OFFICE. THIS was true in the late nineteenth century, and it is true in the early twenty-first. It is the rare physician who can keep track of the torrent of new medical research—and it's even less common to find one who manages to integrate that information into the care he delivers in his office, day in, day out.

Recent research bears this out. In 2000, two data scientists from the University of Missouri, E. Andrew Balas and Suzanne A. Boren, measured the lag from lab to doctor's office by analyzing a handful of common clinical procedures such as mammograms, cholesterol screenings, and flu vaccinations. They tracked when the breakthrough research was first discovered and then worked their way forward, through peer review, publication, into textbooks, and to widespread implementation. The question was, how long did it take? Two years? Five years? A decade?

In fact, Balas and Boren found an average of a seventeen-year delay between the original research establishing a best practice and the time when patients would be routinely treated accordingly. A report issued by the august Institute of Medicine the following year was downright despondent. "Scientific knowledge about best care is not applied systematically or expeditiously to clinical practice. It now takes an average of 17 years for new knowledge generated by randomized controlled trials to be incorporated into practice, and even then application is highly uneven." Seventeen years—it was an astounding finding, one that shook the perception that doctors were practicing scientists fully versed and up-to-date in their disciplines.

The challenge here, what's known as translational medicine, is that clinical doctors must accept the findings of research scientists, a different breed altogether. This requires an idea in one discipline to flow into a related but distinct field, what the theorist Everett Rogers called the "diffusion of innovations." Rogers's book of that title (published, as it happens, in 1962, the same year as Kuhn's *The Structure of Scientific Revolutions*) offers a tidy model for the process. As Rogers describes it, a new innovation doesn't simply erupt into widespread use all at once. Instead, it gradually spreads through a professional class, as some adopt the new tool with enthusiasm, while more reluctant actors sit back and let their peers take the risks and work out the kinks. It's a steady process, but it can be a slow one.

Rogers developed his model by studying how a new weed killer spread among a community of farmers in Story County, Iowa, in the 1950s. Developed by British scientists during World War II to boost production of food crops, the herbicide, known as 2,4-D, is a synthetic plant hormone that causes weeds to, in effect, grow themselves to death. After the war, the chemical made its way to the American Grain Belt, and to Iowa, where Rogers's story starts. First, one farmer (known as Farmer A) heard about the spray through an agricultural researcher. A science enthusiast, Farmer A decided to give it a try, and that year he used it on his corn crop. It worked well for him, and his yield increased substantially—a result keenly observed by Farmer A's neighbor, Farmer B. Within two years, Farmer B had begun using the weed killer, too. Word of the success of Farmer B, who had more stature among the local farmers than Farmer A, spread quickly. The next year, four neighboring farmers adopted the herbicide, and by the following year, five others had as well. After eight years, the last holdouts had signed up to use the spray, and all thirteen farmers in the area had adopted the herbicide.

Though one may not associate 1950s Iowa farmers with the vanguard of technology, their example perfectly illustrates not only how an innovation spreads in terms of time, but the necessary elements for its diffusion as well. Rogers stipulates that four distinct components have to be in place. First is the new technology itself: the new herbicide. The technology is all well and good, Rogers argues, but it is inconsequential without the second component: communication and transmission of its virtues among a possible community of users. In the case of the herbicide, this was, first, the relationship between the scientist and Farmer A, and then, even more significantly in terms of adoption, the relationship between Farmers A and B, who had some influence in the community. Rogers's third element is time, which in this case meant the annual adoption, season by season, by one farmer to the next, as word spread and evidence of the weed killer's effectiveness proved itself. Finally, Rogers notes that an innovation must transition through a coherent social system, a group aligned toward a common goal—in this case, the goal of having a good corn crop that can successfully lead to another one.

The practicality of the herbicide meant that word spread through the network of Iowa farmers rather quickly, all things considered. Within eight years, the entire local community of thirteen farmers was on board with the new spray. Even the laggards (Rogers's term for the latecomers) couldn't deny the success of the herbicide after observing their neighbors' bounty over the past seven years. Indeed, 2,4-D would turn out to be one of the essential agents for the so-called Green Revolution, the massive upswing in farm productivity and food production worldwide made possible by the widespread use of chemical fertilizers and herbicides.

Taken together, Kuhn and Everett offer a framework for the consecutive hoops that a radical idea such as the germ theory would have had to jump through on its way toward general recognition: first acceptance among scientists, then among doctors and physicians, and finally by society at large.

Doctors in the late 1800s weren't so different from those today. The germ theory may have gotten scientists talking, but it had few practical implications, aside from smallpox and anthrax vaccines. Until new discoveries were joined by new treatments, doctors could justifiably sit on the fence. As an 1893 discussion of the germ theory in *The Westminster Review* put it, "the evidence that it is so is powerful and has been accepted by many eminent men of science. The working medical profession as a body have I believe been slower of conviction."

One snag for the germ theory was that, despite the widespread discussion in esteemed journals of Koch's and Pasteur's research, practitioners stubbornly preferred to trust their own clinical experience. Rogers called this homophily—the tendency we all have to seek out like-minded folk. (The aversion to people who are opposed to our beliefs he called heterophily.) This created an additional burden for a novel idea such as the germ theory: Enough opinion leaders and change agents would have to accept the idea and promulgate it before the most determined opponents were convinced of its worth. Or one could simply wait for the old guard to pass and for a new, more accepting generation to come along.

As it happened, the timing was just about perfect for the latter: It had been fourteen years exactly since Lister began publishing on carbolic acid and antiseptic surgery, and twenty since Pasteur's 1861 work debunking spontaneous generation. The time was right for the shift from the theoretical to the practical.

IN SOUTHSEA, CONAN DOYLE CONTINUED TO BUILD HIS MEAGER practice. He arranged for his younger brother, Innes, to join him. He had secured "as nicely furnished a little consulting room as a man need wish to have" and was working on the waiting room. To support himself and his brother, Conan Doyle took on the role as medical examiner for the local Gresham Life Assurance Society, performing autopsies upon request. And he wrote copious letters home to his mother—preferring to use the back side of patients' notes, "as they serve the double purpose of saving paper and of letting you see that business is stirring." He wrote an article on rheumatism for *The Lancet*, though it was never published. For an added bit of cash, he wrote the copy for an advertisement for the Gresham insurance agency, a dour bit of verse, his mind still clearly on germs and infection:

> *When pestilence comes from the pest-ridden South,*
> *And no quarter of safety the searcher can find,*
> *When one is afraid e'en to open one's mouth,*
> *For the germs of infection are borne on the wind.*
> *When fruit it is cheap, and when coffins are dear;*
> *Ah then, my dear friends, 'tis a comfort to know*
> *That whatever betide, we have by our side,*
> *A policy good for a thousand or so.*

> *When the winter comes down with its escort of ills,*
> *Lumbago and pleurisy, toothache and cold;*

When the doctor can scarce with his potions and pills
Keep the life in the young, or death from the old;
When rheumatic winds from each cranny and chink
Seize hold of our joints in their fingers of snow;
Still whatever betide, we retain by our side
That policy good for a thousand or so.

Considering a physician wrote it, the verse affords little promise to medicine. But then, the sad truth was that England in the 1880s would have been a lonely place to aspire to be a man of medicine, regardless.

Consider, first, the state of the art, or what passed for it. Practically speaking, medicine in the 1880s didn't work that well, and routine practices tended to have the opposite of their intended effect. (The one consolation was that most patients' expectations tended to be rather modest.) Even the royalty were vulnerable to the perils of disease, particularly infectious disease. In 1861, Prince Albert, the husband of Queen Victoria, died of typhoid, and a decade later the same disease brought his son the Prince of Wales (later King Edward VII) to the brink of death.

Humoral medicine was still common. The 1862 International Exhibition in London, the greatest display of forward-looking technology in human history up to that time, amazed visitors with stereoscope photography, ice-making machines, and Charles Babbage's "difference engine." But the display of medical equipment featured the latest in leech tubes, lancets, "scarificators," and other bloodletting apparatuses. These instruments looked impressive and modern, in a grisly sort of way, but they were more connected with the Middle Ages, centuries prior, than with the revolutionary research under way in Europe.

And bloodletting was something *real doctors* were offering. There was also a booming industry in flimflam, with healers peddling bogus remedies and ineffective cures. Hydrotherapy was in vogue, constituting various baths at various temperatures for various conditions.

With legitimate pharmacology scarce, hucksters made fortunes selling vegetable pills, Valentine's Meat-Juice, and other "secret" medicines. Homeopathy, the sham practice of using that which causes disease to cure it, was also booming in the 1800s. Despite these quacks, Britain held off from regulating its medical profession until 1858. (France, by contrast, had regulated the practice of medicine since 1794, and Germany, which had long tightly regulated medical practitioners, took the opposite step, in 1869, of loosening the government's hold on practice in order to increase access to care.)

The Lancet and the *BMJ* were both created, in equal parts, to take on the quacks and to undercut the elitism of the Royal College of Physicians. *The Lancet* came first, in 1823, when Thomas Wakley announced the creation of a journal that would hold medicine to high ideals and privilege the pursuit of scientific knowledge. Wakley imagined a new sort of communication channel, both to and from doctors. The *Provincial Medical and Surgical Journal* followed in 1840—it was renamed the *British Medical Journal* in 1888—and likewise endeavored to bring physicians the latest reports and research of medical science. Together, these journals, along with a tide of smaller journals, brought science to an audience hungry for some communication. This new wave promised to wash away inherited practices from the medical profession and allow for an approach steeped in rigor and science.

It's at this point, when new ideas were uprooting the old, that Conan Doyle entered the field—and happily for him, in a place with a focus on the future rather than the past. Edinburgh was a global center of medicine, and a hub of the new *scientific* medicine in particular. It was in Edinburgh where the discovery of chloroform, a powerful anesthetic, had helped initiate the era of modern surgery in 1847. Edinburgh was home to James Syme, the brilliant Scottish surgeon who had led the cause of medical reform in the 1850s that culminated in the Medical Act of 1858. In 1869, Joseph Lister, then just a few years into his work on carbolic acid, replaced Syme as the new chair of clinical surgery. His work on antiseptic surgery was already stirring excitement (and some antipathy) among his peers, and he quickly brought Edinburgh's wards around to his methods. As Conan Doyle described it later, the operations at Edinburgh were "conducted amid clouds of carbolic steam."

Still, inside the lecture halls, there was conflict. The wizened professors scoffed at the germ theory, just as they had disparaged Virchow's cellular pathology a few years earlier. Conan Doyle described these men as "the cold-water school," which regarded "the whole germ theory as an enormous fad." One miffed professor of surgery openly mocked the idea of germs. "Please shut the door, or the germs will be getting in," he scoffed at students.

Conan Doyle quickly aligned himself with the new guard. His most celebrated teacher was Joseph Bell, a professor of surgery who practiced alongside Lister during his stint as chief of surgery in Edinburgh. Bell's approach to germs was more pragmatic than Lister's, abstaining from the philosophical debate but granting the validity of antiseptic methods. In an 1887 book on surgery, Bell made a thoroughly rational assessment: "These germs, they give us anxiety enough, and the practical question we have to settle is, How best to prevent them getting into a wound or harming it after they have got in? We need not greatly care to discuss what is called the germ theory, which some believe in, and some do not; but we may accept it as a valuable idea to keep always before our eyes—the prevention of all infection of a wound."

Bell recruited Conan Doyle as an assistant, and there the latter had a firsthand look at Bell's close powers of observation. "His strong point was diagnosis, not only of disease, but of occupation and character," Conan Doyle would recall. "I had to array his outpatients, make simple notes of their cases, and then show them in, one by one, to the large room in which Bell sat in state surrounded by his dressers and students. Then I had ample chance of studying his methods and of noticing that he often learned more of the patient by a few quick glances than I had done by my questions." Dr. Bell and his talents would make a lifelong impression on Conan Doyle and turn out to be very useful indeed.

And then it was on to Southsea.

In many respects, Conan Doyle and Koch had parallel circumstances: both had made their way from anonymous middle-class circumstances to a local university that, by good grace, was staffed by some of the leading scientists of the day. But after graduation, each had been dispatched to the hinterlands, left to make his own way. And each yearned to make his way back to a place where new ideas were being pursued.

"Let me once get my footing in a good hospital and my game is clear," Conan Doyle wrote his mother during his medical training. "Observe cases minutely, improve my profession, write to the *Lancet*, supplement my income by literature, make friends and conciliate everyone I meet, wait ten years if need be, and then when my chance comes be prompt and decisive in stepping into an honorary surgeonship." As life plans go, it was perhaps not the most ambitious. But Conan Doyle's plan was practical, reasonable, and within reach. As it would happen, it would be both too ambitious in the short term and altogether irrelevant in the long term.

THOUGH THE FIELD OF MEDICINE WAS FAST SHIFTING TOWARD science, the public remained distrusting of the profession. This stemmed from not just ineffective practices, but also ones considered downright depraved. It started with human autopsies.

Cadavers were hard to come by in nineteenth-century England. Until the 1832 Anatomy Act, it was illegal to conduct an autopsy except on a criminal who had been explicitly sentenced to one, following execution. This provided a mere handful of legal corpses annually for several thousand medical students, physicians, and scientists. Given the law of supply and demand, the result, inevitably, was an active black market in bodies. Body snatching became a regular occurrence at English graveyards. After the burial of a loved one, family members routinely took turns at the grave, standing as sentries for several days to keep the body at peace.

Many physicians were willing to ignore the provenance of the corpses they studied—at least until the infamous case of William Burke and William Hare. Sometime in the 1820s, these two Irishmen began supplying fresh corpses to Dr. Robert Knox, a professor at Edinburgh medical school, who needed them to instruct his students, though Knox chose not to ask where the bodies were coming from. Burke and Hare found their supply among the local prostitutes and lodgers in Edinburgh's slums, murdering them for an eight- or ten-pound bounty. By the time they were caught, they had procured at least seventeen corpses for Dr. Knox, who was not prosecuted but fled the city in disgrace, his house burned to the ground. Hare turned king's evidence, and Burke was hanged, but such was the disgust at the case that his body was publicly anatomized and flayed, then skinned, tanned, and sold by the strip. Outrage at the case spurred passage of the Anatomy Act, which required anatomists to obtain a license but allowed them to use any criminal's corpse and allowed individuals to donate a corpse in exchange for the cost of burial.

Even after the Anatomy Act, though, human cadavers remained scarce, and doctors began turning to animals. The use of animals for medical research dates at least as far back as Galen in AD 200. (He based his medical writings on necroscopies of apes and dogs, not humans, a difference that caused centuries of misunderstanding about human anatomy.) But the use of animals took off in the 1840s, with the discovery of cells and the emergence of physiology. As the humoral theory faded, scientists were eager to learn about the function of individual organs, blood vessels and nerves, and other anatomical systems. By the 1870s, the combination of Listerism and anesthesia had made surgery a safer, more viable treatment, increasing the demand for animal stand-ins. And animals (in particular, dogs) were the most available to study systematically.

Simultaneously, laboratory science demanded more animal experiments. As Koch's work with field mice and guinea pigs and Pasteur's experiments with livestock demonstrated, new understanding of the origins and process of disease stemmed directly from animal testing—the germ theory couldn't have existed without them. But as the use of animals for medical research increased, it generated new questions of morality and decency. These questions only grew as it became clear that there were few standards for the treatment or care of animals in these experiments, particularly when it came to vivisection—the dissection of animals while they're still alive.

In part, medical scientists were the victims of a larger failure to reckon with the care of animals, even as society had grown increasingly dependent upon them. Despite its industrial nature, much of the progress of the nineteenth century was borne on the backs of animals, beasts that were as poorly treated as they were indispensable. Indeed, to live in London in midcentury was to be surrounded by animals at every turn. The city's 2.5 million humans lived cheek by jowl with some 300,000 horses and untold hundreds of thousands of pigs, chickens, dogs, cats, and sheep (among the unintended consequences being the mountains of manure they produced, a grave problem for public sanitation).

Even under the best conditions, these animals were in for a rough life. The average life span of a streetcar horse was barely two years. (Horses can typically live twenty-five to thirty years.) In New York, which, like London, was dependent on horses as the engines of commerce and transportation, some fifteen thousand horses died on its streets annually, the victims of beatings, malnourishment, and injury. The misery of these animals was inescapable for city dwellers. In 1824 a group of reformers (led by Richard Martin, a member of Parliament known as "Humanity Dick") formed the Society for the Prevention of Cruelty to Animals, the first charity for animal welfare in the world. Sympathizing with the group, in 1840 Queen Victoria gave it royal sanction.

By the 1860s, animal welfare had become a formidable cross-social movement of Quakers, feminists, popular authors, and reforming politicians. They argued not just against outright cruelty, but that any treatment that jeopardized animals for the advantage of humanity was a crime against nature. This included, quite specifically, the vivisection of animals in scientific experiments. Charles Dickens captured the spirit of the argument in "Inhumane Humanity," an essay published in 1866 in his journal *All the Year Round*. "No doubt it will be said that such experiments are justifiable and necessary in the interests of surgical science for the benefit of mankind. Their necessity I dispute," he wrote. "Man may be justified—though I doubt it—in torturing the beasts that he himself may escape pain. But he certainly has no right to gratify an idle and purposeless curiosity through the practice of cruelty."

The antivivisectionists found their hero in Frances Power Cobbe, a rampaging suffragette and defender of animal rights. The daughter of a leading Anglo-Irish family in Dublin, Cobbe rejected traditional women's roles and devoted herself to religious philosophy and, increasingly, social justice. One of her first attacks on vivisection was an 1863 essay titled "On the Rights of Man and the Claims of Brutes," a vivid description of the horrors of animal experiments conducted in a college of medicine in Paris. In what would become Cobbe's trademark sarcastic tone, she assumed the voice of a mock-biblical epic:

> They took a number of tame and inoffensive animals—but principally those noblest and most sensitive animals, horses— and having bound them carefully for their own safety, proceeded to cut, hew, saw, gouge, bore, and lacerate the flesh, bones, marrow, heart, and brains of the creatures groaning helpless at their feet. And in so orderly and perfect a fashion was this accomplished, that these wise men, and learned men, and honourable men discovered that a horse could be made to suffer for ten hours, and to undergo sixty-four different modes of torture before he died. Wherefore to this uttermost

limit permitted by the Creator did they regularly push their cutting and hacking, delivering each horse into the hands of eight inexperienced students to practise upon him in turn during the ten hours. This, therefore, they did in that great city, not deigning to relieve the pains they were inflicting by the beneficial fluid whereby all suffering may be alleviated, and not even heeding to put out of their agonies at the last the poor mangled remnants of creatures on which they had expended their tortures three score and four.

In 1875, Cobbe founded London's Society for the Protection of Animals Liable to Vivisection; that organization was soon joined by the Victoria Street Society, and that same year the antivivisection cause earned the public support of Queen Victoria. The queen endorsed a Royal Commission on Vivisection in July 1875, and in August 1876, Parliament passed the Cruelty to Animals Act, which prohibited experimentation on animals without the use of anesthetic. The act required scientists to acquire a license for animal experiments but allowed the process and the licensees to remain confidential.

In April 1881, Cobbe turned her artillery squarely on the medical profession in an essay in the popular *Modern Review* titled "The Medical Profession and Its Morality."

Doctors are daily assuming authority which, at first, perhaps, legitimate and beneficial, has a prevailing tendency to become meddling and despotic. . . . It would seem as if our ancestors scarcely realised how painful is sickness, how precious is life—so enhanced is our dread of disease, so desperately anxious are we to postpone the hour of dissolution! As old Selden said, "To preach long, loud, and damnation is the way to be cried up. We love a man that damns us, and run after him to save us." "To preach long, loud and *sanitation*" is the modern doctor's version of this apophthegm, and we do "cry

them up," and run after them to save us from "germs" and all
other imps of scientific imagination.

The mockery of germs as "imps of scientific imagination" was a
trenchant insult. If medicine was a true science, with virtues that
placed it beyond the strictures of society, then where, she scoffed, were
the cures for the "most terrible scourges of mortality, such as cholera,
or consumption, or cancer"? This lack of demonstrable progress, Cobbe
argued, was testimony that, for all their laboratories, physicians should
follow the Victorian rules of decency and humility, like everyone else.

It was a worthy point, touching on the germ theory's greatest vul-
nerability: True or not, what measurable improvement had it fostered
for human health? Cobbe's larger point was valid as well. For decades,
scientific research had been guilty of great cruelty in animal experiments, particularly in those years before Koch and Pasteur began to
establish a clear methodology for experimentation. By 1881, Cobbe's
efforts had succeeded in bringing some decency to the research, and
yet she was not satisfied.

The stakes grew higher when Pasteur had his triumph at Pouilly-
le-Fort in 1881. While a victory for science, Pasteur's experiments had
the consequence of fusing antivivisection with another controversial
scientific practice: the use of vaccines. Vaccines had been controversial
in the United Kingdom since 1853, when Parliament made the
smallpox vaccine compulsory for all newborns. In 1867 the law was
extended to all children fourteen years and younger and assigned
penalties for refusal. Public antipathy to this law was widespread, fed
by the perception that the state was exceeding its authority and in-
vading citizens' homes. Wrote one antivaccination tract, "Are we to
be leeched, bled, blistered, burned, douched, frozen, pilled, potioned,
lotioned, salivated . . . by Act of Parliament?" In London and other
English cities, antivaccination leagues began forming, and periodicals
started to appear, such as *The Vaccination Inquirer,* published by the
London Society for the Abolition of Compulsory Vaccination. The

discoveries of Koch and Pasteur didn't dissuade people from this revolt. Rather, the antivaccination movement found evidence of conspiracy in the rising tide of microbial disease. More germs, the *Inquirer* noted, would inevitably create more vaccines and let the medical establishment continue to perpetrate its witchcraft. Every so-called discovery was just a way for scientists to keep experimenting upon an unwitting and unwilling populace.

The antivaccine movement, of course, was confused by the paradox created by all vaccines: The more effective the vaccine, the more invisible its effectiveness became. The perceived side effects, meanwhile, were readily apparent and easily linked to the trauma of inoculation. To be sure, smallpox vaccines at the time were imperfect. Most vaccinations resulted in at least a fever and occasionally death. Many practicing physicians were sympathetic with the antivaccine crowd; they were themselves concerned about the high rates of illness in children following vaccination, illness that many felt was entirely unnecessary. But the vaccine opponents' argument, by and large, wasn't concerned with whether vaccines represented the greater good. They were opposed outright to the invasion of the sanctity of their bodies, their families, and their rights by a newly aggressive medical profession.

In this, the antivaccination leagues found a common enemy with the antivivisection groups. Both movements were deeply distrustful of the advances in scientific medicine, insofar as these discoveries were used to justify the insult, be it animal experiments or human vaccination. Moreover, the two arguments bore on each other. Antivivisectionists such as Cobbe were deeply skeptical of the argument that vaccines helped prevent disease and, therefore, legitimized animal experiments for the development of such treatments. Cobbe herself claimed that vaccines were more dangerous than the diseases themselves. Denouncing the "vivisecting staffs of Koch and Pasteur," she wrote in her journal, *The Zoophilist,* that "the experiment-intoxicated mind of the medical world cannot be brought to see if this grand prophylactic were adopted, there would soon be an end of epidemics and consumption, for the simple reason that there would be an end of the population."

On some level, the resistance of many British citizens to the incursion of medicine into their homes was understandable. The nineteenth century had seen a series of parliamentary acts that advanced the role of state-sanctioned medicine, at the perceived expense of individual liberty. Beginning with the 1832 Anatomy Act and continuing with the Public Health Act in 1848, the Vaccination Act in 1853, the Contagious Diseases Act in 1864, and the Infectious Diseases (Notification) Acts of 1889 and 1899 (which required the reporting of contagious diseases and confined the sick to hospitals), advances in medicine seemed to be negatively correlated with the autonomy of the common citizen. Time and again, medical science was compelling people to change the way they lived, disrupting norms, and putting notions of public health above those of personal rights. The result was an anti-science libertarianism that took umbrage at an increasingly paternalistic state. At every turn, science was being deployed to constrain the public, a public that was poorly equipped to assess the validity of the science.

This tension, of course, is still palpable today. From the animal rights movement to the antivaccine chorus, from creationists to climate change skeptics, science remains as contentious today as it was in the late nineteenth century, on many of the same issues. As much as science offers the benefits of truth and progress, it often instead generates fear and resistance. This resistance can be readily measured by counting cases of diseases that, given available vaccines, simply shouldn't occur at all. Start with whooping cough, or pertussis. Before a vaccine was developed in the 1940s, it was a major killer of children, with two hundred thousand US cases annually not uncommon. Once the vaccine was widely adopted, though, pertussis was nearly eliminated from the United States. But lackadaisical vaccination, along with the perception that the vaccine was more dangerous than the disease, has caused a resurgence over the past decade, with more than twenty-seven thousand cases in 2010—double the number in 2009. In Europe, where vaccination rates have been plummeting as more governments allow for voluntary immunization, measles has roared back. In 2011 there were nearly thirty thousand cases and a dozen deaths across Europe, three times the number in 2007. (Pasteur would be devastated to know that half these cases occurred in France.)

As in the nineteenth century, the politics of this resistance to science—science that is able readily to reduce illness, eliminate suffering, and save lives—can be confounding. In the United States, for instance, vaccine refusal is frequently widespread in the most affluent, most educated communities, where a combination of presumed sophistication ("I know what's best for my family") along with a distrust of corporate interests (the hostility toward "Big Pharma") can result in parents opting to avoid vaccines. As in the 1880s, a paradox is at work here: Vaccines have been so effective at eliminating the disease they would prevent that the risks of vaccination seem to outweigh the risk of getting the disease.

A century after Koch, in 1990, Carl Sagan, the great popularizer of science, expressed this paradox precisely: "We live in a society exquisitely dependent on science and technology, in which hardly anyone knows anything about science and technology." Science asks people to take a leap of faith. After Jenner developed his smallpox vaccine, for example, people were asked to roll up their sleeves and get vaccinated against something that nobody would thoroughly understand for another seventy-five years. Discoveries forced people to think about how they washed themselves, how they cooked their food, and how they raised their children. Science, in very ordinary terms and very measurable ways, created upheaval.

Science had aroused social controversy before the waning years of the nineteenth century, to be sure. One need only recall Copernicus,

Galileo, and Darwin. But the disputes these earlier thinkers engendered were confined to elites. However controversial they were, the disagreements were largely philosophical, not material. In other words, they infuriated the priests, but the parishioners were too busy working for a living to pay them much mind.

This wasn't at all the case with the scientific controversies of nineteenth-century Europe, and of Britain in particular. Now, for perhaps the first time in human history, scientific discovery was making its way into people's homes, affecting how they conducted the daily business of their lives. To the skeptics, this was more intrusion than they were willing to bear.

ORDINARY DOCTORS SUCH AS CONAN DOYLE FOUND THEMSELVES conscripted into a war that Cobbe and her legions eagerly framed as a battle between science and citizens. For his part, Conan Doyle was plainly frustrated with the anti-science rhetoric and embarrassed for his country. Where scientists were championed as heroes in Berlin and Paris, in England to defend science was to invite mockery and suspicion. Though he was toiling in a tuppence-and-shilling practice in Southsea, he'd learned enough in Edinburgh to grasp the challenge of medical research and the promise it held for human health. He was keenly aware of how much medicine had changed in recent decades and how it had gone from largely palliative to genuinely preventive. His 1883 "Life and Death in the Blood" essay was clearly one gesture at reframing the issue. Out in Europe great men were doing great work. The work of Koch and Pasteur and others, Conan Doyle declared, "has opened up a romance world of living creatures so minute as to be hardly detected by our highest lenses, yet many of them endowed with such fearful properties that the savage tiger or venomous cobra have not inflicted one-fiftieth part of the damage upon the human race." In 1883 he began delivering lectures to the Portsmouth

Literary and Scientific Society and was himself elected to the council a few months in.

He first took up arms—which is to say, his pen—in 1883, to chastise opponents of the Contagious Diseases Act. The law, which was first passed in 1864 and amended in 1866 and 1869, allowed police to arrest prostitutes and subject them to checks for venereal disease. Any woman found to be infected was subject to confinement in a hospital for up to a year. The law was clearly unfairly punitive to the women; their male customers were subject to no such treatment. But in the face of a rising campaign against the law, Conan Doyle felt obliged to speak up and point out the rampant threat to the public health that infectious disease presented. In a letter to *The Medical Times and Gazette,* he argued for the greater good. "For fear delicacy should be offended where no touch of delicacy exists, dreadful evils are to result, men to suffer, children to die, and pure women to inherit unspeakable evils," he lamented. "It becomes a matter of public calamity that these Acts should be suspended for a single day, far more for an indefinite period."

A few years later, it was mandatory vaccination laws that needed defending. After a Col. S. B. Wintle of Southsea objected to vaccination in the local newspaper, Conan Doyle rushed to defend the practice. "The interests at stake are so vital," he wrote in response, "that an enormous responsibility rests with the men whose notion of progress is to revert to the condition of things which existed in the dark ages before the dawn of medical science." After brandishing statistics that showed that the incidence and mortality rate of smallpox were decreasing, he offered a more heartfelt argument to counter Colonel Wintle. "Is it immoral to preserve a child from a deadly disease by methods that have been proven by science and experience?"

Colonel Wintle soon argued back that epidemics of smallpox continued to break out in London and Liverpool. So much for vaccines, he implied. Conan Doyle answered with more evidence: "The death rate varies from less than one in a hundred among the well-vaccinated to the enormous mortality of 37 per cent among Colonel Wintle's followers." He further noted that London and Liverpool both had large transient populations that made it difficult to enforce the vaccination laws fully. Finally, he got personal. Colonel Wintle, like all those who would argue against vaccination, "undertakes a vast responsibility when, in the face of the overwhelming testimony of those who are brought most closely into contact with the disease, he incites others . . . to take their chance of infection in defiance of hospital statistics."

Throughout his life, Conan Doyle would be a fighter, a fierce defender of causes he felt just. In countering the attacks on medicine during the 1880s, and particularly those against the cause of infectious disease, he was convinced that science could bring certainty, that there was precision and definition and *utility* in medicine. Scientific medicine didn't just offer a new way to look at disease—it offered doctors a weapon to combat it. Science made it possible to discern facts out of ambiguity, to give people answers to their questions.

For a medical doctor, this must have been not only exciting, but also something of a relief, considering how often patients knocked on Conan Doyle's door with the hope of a cure but never the expectation of one. Years later, in a speech to medical students, Conan Doyle would recollect the tentative benefits of medical practice. "Someone described our condition as that of a blind man with a club, who swung it at random. Sometimes he hit the disease and sometimes the patient."

In 1885, resolved to improve his career in medicine, Conan Doyle submitted his thesis for his MD. At the time, it was possible to practice medicine with only a bachelor's degree, which Conan Doyle had earned in 1881. Yet the MD was a further mark of respectability, and thus he hoped "those magic letters behind my name" would make him more marketable in Southsea. His chosen topic was the "Vasomotor Changes in Tabes Dorsalis," a degeneration of the nervous system. The disease is now known to be the result of syphilis, but in 1885 the connection between the two was conjectural. Though syphilis was perceived to be an infectious disease, it had not been proven to be one. It was commonly referred to through its contagious origins. Depending on who the perceived agents were, it was called the French disease, the Italian disease, the Polish disease, the British disease, and so on. It would be decades before the true cause, the bacterium *Treponema pallidum*, was identified, and not until penicillin was developed in the 1940s did a treatment become available.

Conan Doyle's thesis would be assessed on its scientific insights, not its literary merits, but he couldn't help but fill the essay with literary flourish. The descriptions of a chronic syphilitic, for instance, showed the close eye of a detective: "His wife calls his attention to the fact that he has developed a squint, or he finds a dimness come over his sight and the lines of his morning paper become blurred & blotted. Very commonly one of his eyelids drop and he finds he cannot raise it. . . . [V]arious little symptoms show him however that the demon which has seized him has not relaxed his grip." With this paper he ably passed and was granted the MD.

However much "that small square of parchment," as he described it to his mother, affected him in 1886, Conan Doyle soon took up his pen and began writing a new tale. And this time, rather than craft another adventure story, he imagined "something fresher and crisper and more workmanlike," something perhaps not so removed from the world of medicine he toiled in daily.

This time, he began to write a story closer to home.

CHAPTER 6

1887 · The Detective

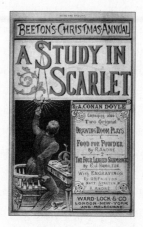

The cover of Beeton's Christmas Annual, *December 1887*

Every November, beginning in 1860, Samuel Beeton, a London publisher, put out a *Christmas Annual,* a collection of stories aimed at the growing English middle class, something families could read together during the holidays. Beeton had made his name, and his fortune, publishing the British edition of *Uncle Tom's Cabin* in 1852, obtaining the rights from Harriet Beecher Stowe before the novel had become an international sensation. His true genius, though, was marrying Isabella Mary Mayson, who, as Mrs. Beeton, would become the phenomenal author of *Beeton's Book of Household Management,* the first reliable cookbook and housekeeping manual. The book launched an empire of self-help guides under Mrs. Beeton's moniker, and Isabella Beeton became one of the first authors to address and exploit the concerns and needs of the domestic British family.

Even though Mrs. Beeton died in 1865, and Samuel Beeton in 1877, the Beeton name endured, under the publishers Ward, Lock and Company, as a proxy for entertaining stories and good, respectable reading material. And in November 1887, the twenty-seventh edition of *Beeton's Christmas Annual* appeared on newsstands in London, at the price of one shilling. The front cover blared out the main story in this year's release: "A Study in Scarlet, by A. Conan Doyle."

Conan Doyle had written the story the previous year, in the spring of 1886, in just six weeks. Several times, he bundled the manuscript up in an envelope and posted it to a publisher, hoping to hook the editors on the unusual tale. But time and again, the manuscript would return to Southsea, sometimes unread, sometimes with a polite note explaining that it just wasn't the sort of thing for their sort of journal. "My poor 'Study,'" Conan Doyle wrote to his mother, "has never even been read by anyone except Payn," referring to the prominent London publisher who had encouraged the young author but who had "found it both too short and too long." Conan Doyle was crestfallen. "Verily literature is a difficult oyster to open. All will come well in time, however."

Among the submissions was one to Ward, Lock and Co., where G. T. Bettany, the chief editor, picked up the manuscript and brought it home. Mrs. Bettany read the story first, and she was smitten. "This is, I feel sure, by a doctor—there is internal evidence," she wrote in a note to her husband. "The writer is a born novelist." In October 1886, Ward, Lock and Co. made an offer: "We have read your story A Study in Scarlet and are pleased with it. We could not publish it this year, as the market is flooded at present with cheap fiction, but if you do not object to its being held over until next year we will give you £25 for the copyright." The fee was meager, the remark about "cheap fiction" was a backhanded compliment, and the request for copyright was an outright insult. Conan Doyle made a counterproposal for royalties, but Ward, Lock refused. Conan Doyle acquiesced. So be it, he thought. Better to have something out under his name in a year than another story stuck in a drawer at 1 Bush Villas.

The offer from Ward, Lock—twenty-five pounds would have been worth about five thousand dollars in today's currency—would help him make a more comfortable home with his new wife, Louise, whom he'd married the previous October. Touie, as Conan Doyle called her, was a quiet, gentle woman of twenty-seven, a year or two older than her new husband. They met under sad circumstances: Louise's brother Jack had come to Dr. Conan Doyle for treatment of his cerebral meningitis caused by infection. Conan Doyle took him in as a resident patient, but he soon died. While coping with her own grief, Louise showed Conan Doyle a good amount of sympathy "for the shock I had suffered, and the disturbance of my household. . . . Before I had spoken to her or knew her name, I felt an inexplicable sympathy for and interest in her." Soon they were married, and she joined Conan Doyle at Bush Villas, offering some sorely needed domestic comforts.

Though it offended him at first, the offer from Ward, Lock was the best he'd had in a good while. Even as his medical practice in Southsea moved along steadily enough, he had begun to worry that his progress in writing was slowing down. "After ten years of such work," he recalled a few years later, "I was as unknown as if I had never dipped a pen in an ink-bottle." His first novel, *The Narrative of John Smith,* had been lost in the mail as it made its way among publishers, and a second, *The Firm of Girdlestone,* was scarcely luckier— not lost, but not published, either. These novels, "written in the intervals of a busy though ill-paying practice," he recalled later, were his effort to rise above the grind of magazine work and affix his name to the spine of a book. Magazine work was frustrating and too anonymous, he believed, the work too quickly lost in the tide of next month's issues. He was beginning to realize that, as he wrote a few years later, "a man may put the very best that is in him into magazine work for years and years, and reap no benefit from it."

He was right to be frustrated. If there was ever a moment for an aspiring writer to taste some success, it was in England in the 1880s. The publishing industry was flourishing, with a staggering amount of reading material streaming off the presses each week. More than 125,000 different periodicals and newspapers were issued in nineteenth-century England, appealing to readers of all stripes. There were bourgeois monthly journals such as *The Pall Mall Gazette, Punch, The Cornhill Magazine*; down-market penny weeklies such as *Tit-Bits* (which had recently rejected Conan Doyle's submission of a Christmas story); and middlebrow sixpenny monthlies such as *Good Words* (where he had published his "Life and Death in the Blood" essay). There were periodicals for suffragists, workmen, boys, and girls. There were so many titles that a new category, the "review," emerged, whose editors would filter the rest of the press to publish a summary of noteworthy articles appearing elsewhere. Some of these, such as *The Edinburgh Review, The Saturday Review*, and *The Fortnightly Review*, became celebrated journals in their own right. Inevitably, there appeared *The Review of Reviews*, offering a further layer of filtering. Meanwhile, there was a cascade of fiction published as cheap books, the novels known as "penny dreadfuls" or "shilling shockers." The Victorian audience consumed them all voraciously.

The explosion of periodicals in the late nineteenth century was fueled by several complementary trends. Costs for producing a newspaper or magazine were dropping as paper production improved, growing train networks enabled cheaper and faster distribution, and printing evolved from a highly manual process to stereotyping. Typesetting, which at the century's beginning required hand-setting, was revolutionized in the 1880s with the linotype machine, which could run entire lines of text at once.

At the same time, literacy rates among the British public were soaring, especially after the 1870 Elementary Education Act provided elementary education for all children, and after compulsory attendance at the board schools (public elementary schools) began to be enforced in the 1880s. These many thousands of periodicals were hungry for words to fill their pages: essays, reporting from across the empire, and the "cheap fiction" produced by those who thought they could spin a tale. Conan Doyle, like many of his contemporaries, saw an opportunity here to be something more. In 1871, some 2,500 Britons identified themselves as writers in the census, five times as many as at the beginning of the century.

In the decade he'd been writing, Conan Doyle had sold a handful of stories, here and there, but *A Study in Scarlet* was his longest piece yet accepted for publication. So he took the Ward, Lock deal. With any luck, if the story was well received, he might return to the character central to *A Study in Scarlet*: an eccentric detective with a surname borrowed from Conan Doyle's favorite physician-philosopher, Oliver Wendell Holmes. He first called him Sherrinford but ultimately settled on something less haughty: Sherlock Holmes. There was something promising about the fellow, Conan Doyle thought. If the public liked Holmes, he might give him another go.

IT'S HARD TO IMAGINE THE WORLD TODAY WITHOUT SHERLOCK Holmes. Holmes has transcended literature to become perhaps the most popular character in Anglo-American culture. In films and television, he remains omnipresent on the scene of contemporary culture, as conspicuous a character as Luke Skywalker or Mickey Mouse. So if we're to appreciate the full breadth of what Conan Doyle created, we must try to push out of our minds everything we think of when we think of Sherlock Holmes and instead consider the vast vacuum of that empty sheet of paper when Conan Doyle sat down at his desk in Southsea and began to sketch out a tale. Originally titled "A Tangled Skein," the story focused on an unlikely duo: this eccentric man with a knack for investigating crime and his newfound acquaintance, a hobbled physician needing a place to live.

It's tempting to slot Conan Doyle into the myth of the lone genius

here, just as it was to consider Koch as such. But just as Koch's
work owed much, in fact, to Henle, Pasteur, and others, so Conan
Doyle's creation can be traced quite clearly to specific influences that
broached even distant Southsea. This first Sherlock Holmes novel
resourcefully cobbled together a range of influences and sources. In
terms of the detective himself, the most obvious predecessor is Edgar
Allan Poe's detective, C. Auguste Dupin. Poe's "The Murders in
the Rue Morgue," published in 1841, is considered the first modern detective story. Conan Doyle devoured the tale as a child and admired it
as an adult. Like Holmes, Dupin relies on logic and intellect more
than happenstance. And like Holmes, Dupin doesn't have an official
position as a detective (a word that hadn't, in any event, been invented
in 1841). He is simply motivated by an urge to put his wits to work, to
wield his powers of reasoning and analysis to do something useful.

Though Conan Doyle clearly drew on Poe, he was also tapping
into a popular enthusiasm for tales of crime and intrigue. By the time
Sherlock Holmes came around, mysteries had been a staple of English
fiction for more than a century. The cascade of periodicals created a
new demand for adventure stories tinged with a bit of criminality. The
novels of Wilkie Collins—first serialized in Charles Dickens's *All the
Year Round* in the 1850s and '60s—invented many of the classic touch-
stones of the genre, such as a local police investigator in over his head,
a handful of false suspects, and the surprise twist.

But Conan Doyle turned out something that, even in the first
appearance in *A Study in Scarlet*, went far beyond his influences. (For
instance, though today many consider his London a definitive portrait
of the city, in fact, Conan Doyle had little firsthand experience in
London and, as he later confessed, had leaned heavily on a post office
map to describe the city in his early Holmes stories.) Sherlock Holmes
wasn't a stock character but had a singular personality and appeal and
a wholly modern approach to his task of criminal detection. "I had
been reading some detective stories, and it struck me what nonsense

they were, to put it mildly, because for getting the solution to the mystery the authors always depended on some coincidence," Conan Doyle explained a few years later in the *Westminster Gazette*. "This struck me as not a fair way of playing the game, because the detective ought really to depend for his successes on something in his own mind and not on merely adventitious circumstances which do not, by any means, always occur in real life." Instead of coincidence, Holmes made his way through keen observation and an idiosyncratic cabinet of knowledge. He was, as first described in *A Study in Scarlet*, "a little queer in his ideas—an enthusiast in some branches of science. . . . His studies are very desultory and eccentric, but he has amassed a lot of out-of-the-way knowledge which would astonish his professors."

Indeed, to read the first Holmes story today is to note how different the detective is, on first appearance, from the omnipotent genius we think of today. In fact, his expertise is erratic and spotty, not broad and deep. His new roommate, Dr. John Watson, is struck by this and describes it at length.

His zeal for certain studies was remarkable, and within eccentric limits his knowledge was so extraordinarily ample and minute that his observations have fairly astounded me. . . . His ignorance was as remarkable as his knowledge.

Of contemporary literature, philosophy and politics he appeared to know next to nothing. Upon my quoting Thomas Carlyle, he inquired in the naivest way who he might be and what he had done. My surprise reached a climax, however, when I found incidentally that he was ignorant of the Copernican Theory and of the composition of the Solar System. That any civilized human being in this nineteenth century should not be aware that the earth travelled round the sun appeared to be to me such an extraordinary fact that I could hardly realize it.

Holmes does not, quite profoundly, *know* everything. Rather, he knows how to gather and assess evidence, to treat a crime scene like an experiment in progress. He knows how to *diagnose* a crime scene. It is his method that makes him singular. It is his process, his thoroughness—and most of all, his ability to connect small observations with a larger body of knowledge, a process that Holmes calls, famously, "the science of deduction."

To contemporary audiences, this flair for discovery was Holmes's most impressive attribute, and it remains his signature trait—and it comes right out of Conan Doyle's experience at Edinburgh. When Conan Doyle served as assistant to Joseph Bell, he witnessed how nimble were Dr. Bell's powers of observation and diagnosis. Conan Doyle would later remember one episode when a new patient arrived, and Bell quickly identified him, apparently without any prior knowledge, as a noncommissioned officer discharged from his Highland regiment stationed in Barbados. Conan Doyle was astonished, but it was entirely obvious, Bell explained: "The man was a respectful man, but did not remove his hat. They do not in the army, but he would have learned civilian ways had he been long discharged. He has an air of authority and he is obviously Scottish. As to Barbados, his complaint is elephantiasis, which is West Indian and not British."

It's an episode that neatly parallels one in *A Study in Scarlet,* when Sherlock Holmes identifies a man walking by on Baker Street as a retired sergeant of the Royal Marines. Watson is sure Holmes is guessing, but when the man rings the doorbell to deliver a package, Watson asks him about his background and is left incredulous when Holmes is proven right. "How in the world did you deduce that?" Watson asks, and Holmes proceeds to tick off the catalog of clues.

For Conan Doyle, Bell's talent for connecting seemingly random clues with a storehouse of knowledge, the way he applied scientific analysis to routine matters, was just the sort of ingenious skill that might turn a stock detective into something more compelling. As he noted later, "I thought I would try my hand at writing a story where the hero would treat crime as Dr. Bell treated disease." In an essay published with a reissue of *Scarlet* a few years later, Bell himself praised how his former student had put his medical training to use. "Dr. Conan Doyle's education as a student of medicine taught him how to observe, and his practice, both as a general practitioner and a specialist, has been a splendid training for a man such as he is, gifted with eyes, memory, and imagination."

Conan Doyle echoed the thought years later speaking to medical students, acknowledging the benefits of medical training. "It tinges the whole philosophy of life and furnishes the whole basis of thought," he said. "The healthy skepticism which medical training induces, the desire to prove every fact, and only to reason from such proved facts— these are the finest foundations for all thought." The words could have been spoken by Sherlock Holmes himself.

SCIENCE RUNS DEEP IN SHERLOCK HOLMES STORIES, AND AS MUCH as that reflects Conan Doyle's background, it also reflects the age. Despite the labors of antivivisectionists and antivaccinationists, despite the denials of those who refused to grant the existence of germs, despite the doubters of Darwin, science was soaring in the last quarter of the nineteenth century. It was the most potent force in European culture, revealing invisible worlds and offering new ways to see the visible world. Electricity arrived in 1873, first with the discovery of electromagnetism, and soon thereafter with a series of inventions with profound cultural implications: 1876 brought the invention of the telephone; 1877 brought Thomas Edison's phonograph; 1879, Edison's incandescent lamp. Cash registers, dishwashers, fountain pens, and the internal combustion engine were all soon to follow.

The pace of progress amazed even chroniclers of science. *The Popular Science Monthly*, founded in New York in 1872, editorialized in 1890, "We have frequent cause for astonishment at the rapidity with which modern life is being transformed under the influence of scientific invention and discovery. . . . The telephone makes its way everywhere without pause or check, and the same is true of electric lighting and traction."

The revolution wasn't just one of household conveniences. All at once, civilization seemed to break free from centuries of tradition and secondhand wisdom and emerge into the bright light of ascertainable truth. Increasingly there was a sense that science was no longer just a tally of things people could now understand, the province of Isaac Newton and the Royal Society; rather, it was a *method,* an approach to the natural world that could be deployed to address a broad range of social problems, from poverty to education to disease. With the scientific method as a weapon, researchers and inventors might tackle any outstanding riddle of the ages and, in short order, produce a solution, an answer. A remedy.

How does a scientific revolution build toward social change? This is perhaps the central question of the past 150 years, a period when science has, time and again, transcended a eureka moment in the laboratory to compel a broader cultural shift. This trajectory lies behind everything from nuclear energy to plastics to the Internet. But as essential as this trajectory is to the fabric of our daily lives, the process too often slips by without our noting it, or even our knowing *how,* precisely, the progress actually happens.

The germ theory is one of history's most vivid examples of this trajectory, rising from Koch's work in Wöllstein to immunology to antibiotics to a new understanding of cancer and heart disease. Along the way, the germ theory also demonstrated what standards of evidence society, rather than scientists, required. In fact, it's worth burrowing a little deeper into the process here, in order to spell out the stages from science to society, in order both to better grasp the consequence of Koch's work and to better understand the role that Conan Doyle, as one sympathetic to science, played.

Both Koch and Sherlock Holmes viewed science as a tool, an

instrument with impact. Freeman Dyson, the Princeton physicist and mathematician, has made this case most emphatically, pointing to astronomy (where the telescope was the revolutionary force) and genetics (where the discovery of the structure of DNA in 1953 is only now being exploited with miniaturized sequencing and synthesis technologies). Science, Dyson argued, generates "unpredictable new ideas and opportunities. And human beings will continue to respond to new ideas and opportunities with new skills and inventions. We remain toolmaking animals, and science will continue to exercise the creativity programmed into our genes."

Dyson's emphasis on tools, it needs to be acknowledged, is a direct refutation of Thomas Kuhn's concept-based theory of science. Where Kuhn argues that science is the progress from revolutionary idea to idea, Dyson insists that the revolution lives in the industry, not the idea. But they're both useful concepts. If Kuhn helps us understand how revolutionary ideas such as the germ theory gain primacy among scientists, Dyson helps us see how such a theory leads to technologies that have profound cultural impact.

In our technology-saturated twenty-first century, it's easy to grasp the powerful simplicity of Dyson's idea. It's manifest in the way we read about science in the newspaper, with today's physics discovery becoming tomorrow's amazing microprocessor. But this transformation of science into technology and technology into cultural change was altogether novel in the 1880s. The profusion of new gizmos, from typewriters to player pianos, was unprecedented. As T. H. Huxley, a celebrated English biologist known as "Darwin's bulldog," wrote in 1866, science had enabled the invention of the great ships crossing the ocean and the railroad crossing the landscape; it had born an infrastructure of factories and printing presses, "without which the whole fabric of modern English society would collapse into a mass of stagnant and starving pauperism." Suddenly, science *mattered;* it was something people wanted to know about, to keep pace with, and to understand.

The editors of thousands of periodicals recognized science as something that had appeal for readers. Science journals, including *Nature* (founded in 1869), bridged the intellectual gap between the publications for scientists and those for lay readers. Book publishers also jumped into the game with scientific primers for general readers: the Nature Series, the Contemporary Science Series, the Manuals of Elementary Science, and dozens more. These publications aimed to popularize science, to make its discoveries evident and comprehendible to all.

In *A Study in Scarlet*, Conan Doyle touches on this enthusiasm in the popular press when Watson picks up a magazine and reads an essay titled "The Book of Life." Though Watson doesn't realize it, the essay is by Holmes. Science, Holmes's essay argues, can yield profound insights simply by reasoning from one point of evidence to the next. "From a drop of water a logician could infer the possibility of an Atlantic or a Niagara without having seen or heard of one or the other. So all life is a great chain, the nature of which is known whenever we are shown a single link of it. . . . By a man's finger nails, by his coat-sleeve, by his boot, by his trouser knees, by the callosities of his forefinger and thumb, by his expression, by his shirt cuffs—by each of these things a man's calling is plainly revealed."

Though Watson dismisses the essay as "ineffable twaddle," Holmes's argument draws from legitimate science. Darwin serves as one example, but there are others. In 1839 the British naturalist Richard Owen was presented with a scrap of bone found in New Zealand. Remarking on its resemblance to an ostrich bone, he conjectured that giant flightless birds once lived in New Zealand. A few years later, he was able to confirm his theory with a skeleton of the ancient moa bird. Similarly, in 1863, T. H. Huxley explained in a widely circulated lecture how French naturalist Georges Cuvier had been able to reconstruct "entire animals from a tooth or perhaps a fragment of bone."

Holmes was working from the same playbook, as Conan Doyle makes clear in "The Five Orange Pips," a later Holmes adventure. "As

Cuvier could correctly describe a whole animal by the contemplation of a single bone, so the observer who has thoroughly understood one link in a series of incidents should be able to accurately state all the other ones, both before and after," Holmes explains.

But Conan Doyle looked not just at science broadly, but at microbiology specifically. The work of Louis Pasteur and, even more so, Robert Koch provided the template for Sherlock Holmes's fascination with minuscule detail.

IF CONAN DOYLE'S EPIPHANY WAS TO TURN LABORATORY ANALYTICS toward real-world problems, there were few concerns more acute for Victorian England than crime. Particularly in London, crime seemed to seep through every neighborhood, oozing throughout the city streets as steadily as slaughterhouse canals and sewers drained into the Thames. The bounty of words for "criminals" gives a sense of the scale of the problem. There were *maltoolers* and *cly fakers, flimps* and *dippers* (all pickpockets), *macers* and *magsmen* (cheats), *dragsmen* and *sharpers* and *buttoners* and *gonophs* (varieties of thieves), and *nobblers* and *bludgers* (violent criminals who might use chloroform to knock out a victim before robbing him). At night, "mutchers" would go "bug hunting" (robbing drunks), or they'd bash a citizen with a "holy water sprinkler" (a cudgel spiked with nails). The 1850s and '60s saw panic over garrotting, with victims being jumped from behind, a rope drawn across their throats. Even children were at risk, as well-dressed youths would be pulled into alleys and stripped of their clothes. (Poor children were organized into gangs of pickpockets by criminals known as kidsmen, à la Fagin in *Oliver Twist*.) Prostitution was rampant, most prominently in theater alleys and along the banks of the Thames— not coincidentally, places that also were frequented by thugs waiting to rob a would-be customer. The prostitutes themselves were inevitably at risk as well, as the five brutal murders attributed to Jack the Ripper brought to light in 1888.

Whether the streets were, in fact, growing more dangerous was unclear to many Londoners. The Metropolitan Police was founded in London in 1829, though the force was for decades afflicted by drunkenness, ineptitude, and corruption. At best, some fourteen hundred police officers patrolled daily over a population greater than five million. Certainly, the rise of media helped fuel a sense of lawlessness. During the garroting panics, from 1855 to 1860, the circulation of daily newspapers increased threefold.

In fact, crime may have been going down by the time Sherlock Holmes appeared on the scene, at least according to the statistics available. In the 1860s there were six property felonies for every 1,000 Londoners, but by the late 1880s that rate had fallen to 2.5 per 1,000 citizens. Violent crimes fell similarly, despite the headlines generated by the Ripper murders. Though crime was still greatly feared in London and elsewhere, it no longer seemed the inevitable ulcer of a much deeper cultural corruption. By the late 1880s, the topic of crime didn't provoke despair so much as action. There was increasingly a sense that crime could be fought and criminals prosecuted.

This was the spirit that Conan Doyle brought to the subject, and it was a key appeal to his Sherlock Holmes. Rather than offer one more stock detective who stumbled his way through a crime, Conan Doyle gave Holmes a way to assess it, scrutinize it, and attack it. Holmes puts science to work, revealing clues others miss. He demonstrates that crime is no match for science.

And notably Holmes doesn't just *apply* science to crime solving; he develops it himself. Holmes makes his first appearance at 221b Baker Street in his makeshift lab, with a test tube in hand. "I've found it! I've found it!" he exclaims.

I have found a re-agent which is precipitated by hoemoglobin, and by nothing else.... Criminal cases are continually hinging upon that one point. A man is suspected of a crime months perhaps after it has been committed. His linen or clothes are examined, and brownish stains discovered upon them. Are they blood stains, or mud stains, or rust stains, or fruit stains, or what are they? That is a question which has puzzled many an expert, and why? Because there was no reliable test. Now we have the Sherlock Holmes test, and there will no longer be any difficulty.

In truth, it would be nearly twenty years before the "Sherlock Holmes test"—known as the Kastle-Meyer test—would be able to identify bloodstains accurately. But Holmes's enthusiasm shows Conan Doyle's passion for applying science to crime solving and for the science of criminology just emerging all over Europe, often with specious claims. In Italy, Cesare Lombroso argued that criminals were a racially distinct class of savages and that they could be identified by a taxonomy of physical characteristics. In France, Alphonse Bertillon unveiled what he called "anthropometry," a system for classifying criminals by their physical appearance, tattoos, and scars. More practically, Bertillon advocated taking two photographs of a suspect, in both frontal and profile portraits—inventing what we recognize today as the mug shot.

In *Nature* in 1880, a Scottish physician named Henry Faulds had noted "skin furrows of the hand," particularly on the fingertips. These patterns, he reckoned, seemed to be unique to individuals, leading Faulds to speculate upon their value: "When bloody finger-marks or impressions on clay, glass, etc., exist, they may lead to the scientific identification of criminals."

Though it would be several decades before fingerprints became a standard tool of police work—they first appeared in a 1903 Sherlock Holmes story "The Adventure of the Norwood Builder"—Faulds's insight aligned with the methods that Conan Doyle bequeathed to his fictional detective. In *Scarlet*, for instance, Holmes explains to Watson how footprints might be analyzed, identifying not only a suspect's shoe but his weight and height as well. "There is no branch of detective science which is so important and so much neglected as the art of tracing footsteps," he suggests.

Regardless of whether Conan Doyle was anticipating forensic science or simply keeping up with its pioneers, he created in Sherlock Holmes a textbook demonstration of how to put science to work. In this, the stories seem ideally suited to their historical moment, when science was recognized as a force for good and when the public was hungry for stories that reflected their increasingly modern world. What is surprising to realize today, then, is that when Sherlock Holmes did first appear, he was paid so little notice.

CONAN DOYLE HAD LET HIMSELF HOPE THAT *A STUDY IN SCARLET* would be a triumph, the story that would make his name. Instead, it barely registered.

"I had high hopes," Conan Doyle wrote in his memoirs, confessing that he had imagined that "my little Holmes book" would change his lot. But although it "attracted some favourable comment, the door still seemed to be barred." For the moment, at least.

After *A Study in Scarlet* appeared and disappeared in 1887, Conan Doyle went back to his desk at Bush Villas and resolutely began work on another novel, this one more ambitious and more deliberately literary than anything he had done previously. This was his historical novel *Micah Clarke*. Set in the seventeenth century, it was an adventure story in the style of Sir Walter Scott. Conan Doyle thought it was the best thing he'd ever written (and indeed he would long consider it his best work). Even before it was published, he was already dreaming about how it might allow him to move forward in his life. If it succeeds, he wrote to his sister, "we may then, I think, take it as proven that I can live by my pen. We should have a few hundreds in hand to start us. The next step would be to quietly sell the practice"— the first admission that he wanted out of medical practice. He imagined that he might tour Europe (Berlin, Paris, Vienna), studying ophthalmology, and at last return to London to "start as an eye surgeon, still of course keeping literature as my milk cow."

"But of course all this is mere dreamland tho' it may take shape," he acknowledged. "All depends on Micah."

Micah Clarke was published in February 1889, and it earned more than forty reviews, most of them favorable. Conan Doyle dutifully bought each newspaper and magazine that featured a mention of the book, clipped out the reference, for good or ill, and pasted it into a notebook. But "it was not a boom book," as Conan Doyle later admitted. There was no quitting Southsea, at least not yet, and there was certainly no quitting medicine.

The novel did enable him finally to sell another novel, *The Firm of Girdlestone*, which had languished in a desk drawer for two years. Things turned brighter still when, on August 30, Conan Doyle received an invitation from Joseph Stoddart, the American publisher of *Lippincott's Monthly Magazine*, to have dinner in London. Conan Doyle "gave my patients a rest for a day" and headed to the city. At the appointed hour, he showed up at the grand Langham hotel and was pleased to see that Stoddart had also invited another writer, Oscar Wilde. At the time, Wilde was best known for his witty journalism, his essays on the arts, and his fashion élan. Five years older than Conan Doyle, he was most definitely a *writer,* someone dedicated to the craft, which was more than Conan Doyle could claim.

The dinner went splendidly; Wilde mentioned that he had read *Micah Clarke* and enjoyed it—a tremendous boost to Conan Doyle's ego. Stoddart was impressed by both writers, and he ended the evening by commissioning each of them to write short novels of "not less than 40,000 words." The fee would be a hundred pounds, more than Conan Doyle had earned with his writing the entire year previous. "It was indeed a golden evening for me," Conan Doyle wrote.

Wilde's contribution would be *The Picture of Dorian Gray,* his only novel, and one that would scandalize Victorian London with its thinly veiled homoeroticism and amoral hero. For his part, Conan Doyle had the idea to "give Sherlock Holmes of *A Study in Scarlet* something else to unravel." He took just two months to dash off his effort, *The Sign of Four.*

The short novel, published in the United States and the United Kingdom in February 1890, was controversial in its own right, opening with a scene of Holmes languidly injecting a 7 percent solution of cocaine into an arm already scarred with "innumerable puncture marks." Even more than *Scarlet,* the story is suffused with science, starting with the title of the first chapter, "The Science of Deduction." (This is also the title of chapter 2 in *Scarlet;* the author assumed that many of his readers would be meeting Holmes for the first time.) "Detection," Holmes tells Watson, "is, or ought to be, an exact science and should be treated in the same cold and unemotional manner."

The story abounds in laboratory work and medical references: Heart disease, hypochondria, malaria, and addiction all make an appearance. Holmes informs Watson that he has published several scientific monographs, "all upon technical subjects," from the 140 types of tobacco ash to the influence of a trade upon the form of a hand, "a matter of great practical interest to the scientific detective." This is where Holmes first offers his precept "When you have eliminated the impossible, whatever remains, *however improbable,* must be the truth."

The Sign of Four was well reviewed; *The Daily Telegraph* praised "the excellence of its style [and] the intense interest of its plot." Wilde himself wrote Conan Doyle to praise the "strength and sincerity" of the book. More significantly, in October he received a letter from Lawson Tait, one of Britain's most prominent surgeons. Conan Doyle had only heard of Tait, and he never imagined Tait would reach out himself to write a fan letter. Though we don't have the letter, we do have Conan Doyle's proud description of it to his mother: "He said that He and Lord Coleridge were both great admirers of my 'Study in Scarlet' and of my 'Sign of Four.' He spoke in the kindest way of them." Accolades from Lord Coleridge were a special bonus; the poet's grandnephew, Coleridge was one of the nation's great solicitors, with the rank of lord chief justice of England. If Conan Doyle thought he was toiling in obscurity, suddenly here were twin endorsements from the most accomplished of Britons. It was just the boost in confidence that he needed, and a keen validation of his technique.

At this point, Conan Doyle had been in Southsea for eight years and had been writing stories for a decade. He was happy enough, as he'd recall later in his memoirs. "My life had been a pleasant one with my steadily-increasing literary success, my practice, which was enough to keep me pleasantly occupied, and my sport" (Conan Doyle was an ardent amateur athlete).

But in November 1890, while making notes on proofs of his latest novel, *The White Company,* Conan Doyle took a break and picked up the day's mail. Amid the bills and correspondence was a special supplement to the *British Medical Journal,* published that day: Friday, November 15. Curious as to what would require such a rare dispatch, Conan Doyle began reading.

The report consisted of an update by Robert Koch, the brilliant German bacteriologist. Back in August, at the Tenth International Medical Congress in Berlin, Koch had hinted at a remarkable finding, greater perhaps than the sum of all his previous discoveries. This new dispatch, translated in the *BMJ* from a just-published German article, elaborated on that research. Now Koch explained in detail what he'd alluded to at the congress: He believed he had discovered nothing less than "a remedy which conferred on the animals experimented upon an immunity against inoculation with the tubercle bacillus, and which arrested tuberculous disease," Koch wrote. "There is no question of a destruction of the tubercle bacilli in the tissues." The *BMJ* reported that there would be a public demonstration of Koch's remedy in Berlin on November 17—just two days away. Every medical man of caliber in the world would be there.

As was evident from his "Life and Death in the Blood" essay, Conan Doyle was already a great admirer of Koch's talents. The two men were, in many ways, accidental partners in a profound social shift toward science and away from superstition. Where Koch had proven the merits of science and outlined the methodology, Conan Doyle had put it into action, placing it in the hands of an odd, cantankerous, and rigorous detective who was peculiarly gifted at scientific analysis, to great result. Robert Koch's postulates were not so different from Sherlock Holmes's science of deduction: Both demanded a close analysis of the facts, an absolute fidelity to the truth, and a faith that, properly followed, the process would bring desired results. Both men, after all, swore by the same weapon: the microscope (the instrument shows up in more Holmes stories than even the now-iconic magnifying glass).

In his memoirs, Conan Doyle tells what happened next: "A great urge came upon me suddenly that I should go to Berlin."

> I could give no clear reason for this, but it was an irresistible impulse and I at once determined to go. Had I been a well-known doctor or a specialist in consumption it would have been more intelligible, but I had, as a matter of fact, no great interest in the more recent developments of my own profession, and a very strong belief that much of the so-called progress was illusory. However, at a few hours' notice I packed up a bag and started off alone upon this curious adventure.

If he were to make it to Berlin in time, he would have to leave at once. He quickly informed Touie of his plans, kissed his daughter, Mary, good-bye, and raced to the Portsmouth Station to catch the next train to London. An hour later, the train arrived in Waterloo Station, and Conan Doyle dashed to Mowbray House, headquarters of *The Review of Reviews*. The *Review* was edited by W. T. Stead, with whom Conan Doyle had corresponded the prior year. Although Conan Doyle showed up unannounced, Stead invited him into his office.

Conan Doyle explained to Stead what was about to happen in

Berlin in less than two days. Stead asked why Conan Doyle, of all people, should be the one to cover the demonstration for the *Review*. Conan Doyle explained that, as both a writer and a physician, he was uniquely suited for the job. He could both assess the credibility of Koch's remedy and write up an engaging account of the stakes. Stead was impressed with Conan Doyle's panache and told him that he had intended, himself, to write a medical piece, on Count Mattei, a proponent of electrohomeopathy, for the next issue. The two essays, Stead thought, might complement each other. On the spot, he commissioned Conan Doyle to write a profile of Koch and quickly dashed off both a letter of assignment and one of introduction, to the British ambassador in Berlin, should Conan Doyle need some official assistance.

Conan Doyle was thrilled. He raced out of the office and dashed down Norfolk Street, headed to Victoria Station. He took the next train down to the coast, then hopped a ferry across the Channel. By the next morning, November 16, he was on the Continental Express, rolling toward Berlin's Central Station.

1890 · The Remedy

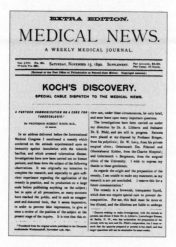

A special edition of the American journal Medical News, *November 15, 1890*

The triumph of discovering the cause of tuberculosis in 1882 stoked something in Robert Koch, an ambition that would have been inconceivable just a few years before in Wöllstein. This was not Koch's better angel; it was the same beast that had attacked Pasteur in 1881 and kept at it during the months of poisonous exchanges. He was now quite unlike the meek hobbyist who had humbly asked Dr. Cohn to check over his kitchen-sink experiments just a few years earlier.

The competition with Pasteur came to a head in the spring of 1883, when a pandemic of cholera began to race across Asia, erupting first in its endemic home of India and then spreading to Turkey and into North Africa. When the outbreak reached Egypt, European countries began to get nervous. This was the latest of several waves of cholera to break out in the nineteenth century, each time spreading misery and death across Europe. The most recent pandemic had only just relented in the late 1870s, a decadelong outbreak that killed more than a million worldwide, including 113,000 in Italy, 165,000 in Austria, 90,000 in Russia, and 30,000 pilgrimaging Muslims in Mecca. There seemed every reason to expect that the disease was now following a similar course. The difference, though, was that in 1875, the germ theory was still speculation; by 1883, however, microbes had been definitively established to cause several diseases. Cholera seemed certain to be next.

Egypt was particularly hospitable to the disease. Most of the country's population was crowded into Cairo and the Nile Delta, dense and dirty communities where sanitation was nonexistent. The major source of water in the country was the Nile, where the clothes of cholera victims were routinely washed. Downstream, the same water was used for drinking. The outbreak followed the classic epidemiological pattern of gaps and clusters, with some towns spared the disease entirely, while others were devastated. Of the 14,000 inhabitants of Shibin el Kom, a village in the Nile Delta north of Cairo, nearly 2,000 were sickened, and fully one in ten died of the disease in just a few weeks. As the summer stretched on, the national death toll climbed quickly, with nearly 6,000 dead in Cairo alone.

In late July, a desperate Egyptian government requested the help of both France and Germany in identifying the cause of the epidemic. In France, the call went to Louis Pasteur, who remained in Paris but dispatched a team of his most able assistants, including Louis Thuillier. The Germans offered Koch, who quickly made arrangements with his home and lab and then left for Egypt, leading Georg Gaffky and three others. The race was on.

The French team, known as "Le Mission Pasteur," arrived in Alexandria first, on August 15, 1883, and found quarters in l'Hôpital Européen, the city's finest medical facility. Koch's team arrived ten days later and set up in the city's Greek Hospital.

For Koch, this was a welcome head-to-head contest against his French rival: one disease, one country, two teams. Fresh from the triumph of his tuberculosis discovery, Koch thought his laboratory precision held the upper hand against the French team's more shotgun-style approach to microbe detection. Within a month, Koch had identified one characteristic organism in several cholera victims; he failed to culture the microbe, nor could he produce an infection in mice, but he was hopeful he was on the right path and published a preliminary but inconclusive report. But just then, the epidemic began to wane, making further experiments impossible. "Cholera has almost disappeared in Alexandria," he soon wrote Emma, "which for our purposes is too early. . . . I am afraid we are without either cholera patients or cholera victims."

The French team, meanwhile, had gotten hold of more cadavers and was still working. It had isolated several different bacteria but couldn't be certain that any one might be causal. But the team did suggest that some "tiny bodies" in blood smears of cholera victims might somehow be involved. (Later Koch would insinuate that the French team had simply found blood platelets.)

On the morning of September 18, Thuillier, the lead French scientist, had a bout of diarrhea. He walked over to a colleague's room. "I feel very ill," he said, then swooned and crumpled to the floor. His alarmed colleagues picked him up, carried him to his bed, and gave him a dose of opium. He seemed to recover slightly but then had what Émile Roux, his fellow team member, described as "a copious watery stool"—the telltale sign of cholera. Thuillier said he felt cold; his legs began cramping. Despite frantic measures, including iced champagne and injections of ether, he died on the morning of the nineteenth. He was twenty-seven years old.

The death was a shock to both teams. A comrade in arms in the battle against microbes had succumbed, a risk that everyone, French or German, knew he faced. Koch and his colleagues hastened over to l'Hôpital Européen and offered their respects. At the funeral, Koch himself served as a pallbearer. The French team left for Paris soon after, its mission incomplete.

Koch, though, was not yet done. With the outbreak all but over in Egypt, he requested permission from the German government, which was funding the expedition, to hunt the disease at the source: India. On November 13, the Germans left Suez en route to Calcutta, home of the Ganges River, which they believed to be the headwaters of the microbe. Once there, Koch spent two months holed up in the Medical College and Hospital, hunched over microscopes and avoiding the stifling heat outside. Despite his being halfway around the world, Koch's progress was surprisingly public: His regular dispatches to the health minister in Berlin were printed in full in German newspapers, reports that were then excerpted and translated in the *BMJ*. Laying out his progress step by step, the dispatches chronicled his methods with characteristic exactitude.

In Calcutta, Koch had plenty of organisms to study. His first material came from a twenty-two-year-old man who had died just ten hours after first showing symptoms; he was only three hours out of autopsy when his intestines were harvested for Koch's investigation. By early February, Koch was confident he'd found the germ, a comma-shaped bacillus that was, finally, growing actively in culture. But he continued to test and retest his results, interrogating his own conclusions until he'd isolated the organism in twenty-two corpses and seventeen living patients. "In all cases," he wrote in his report, "the comma bacillus and only the comma bacillus has been found. These results, taken together with those obtained in Egypt, prove that we have found the pathogen responsible for cholera."

To his frustration, Koch was still unable to transfer the disease successfully to animals, failing to satisfy his own criterion for true causality. Instead, he took a page from John Snow and made a map of the water tanks in one neighborhood where seventeen had recently died. The homes of the deceased formed a neat ring around the tank, not just the source of drinking water in the neighborhood but also a place for bathing and doing laundry. Even the clothes of the cholera victims had been washed in the tank, a sure way to keep the disease active in the neighborhood. His investigation was complete, and on April 4, 1884, he and his team headed home. It would be a brutal trip: Koch would suffer a bout of malaria, forcing a long detour to Cairo. On May 2 he arrived home in Berlin, nearly nine months after he'd left.

"WELCOME VICTORS!" hailed the front page of the *Berliner Tageblatt* on May 3. Koch was received by the kaiser and met with Otto von Bismarck, the imperial chancellor of Germany, who bestowed on him a medal. The celebration culminated in a banquet with seven hundred guests. The program celebrated Koch's expedition as a quasi-military victory, with allusions toward the Franco-Prussian War. "Just as 13 years ago the German people celebrated a glorious victory against the hereditary enemy of our nation, so does German Science today celebrate a brilliant triumph over one of humanity's most menacing enemies." Koch himself was hailed as a national hero and anointed Germany's finest scientist. "In less than a decade, he presented to the world an amazing array of discoveries," one speaker proclaimed, tallying Koch's quarry of anthrax, tuberculosis, and now cholera.

Koch loved every bit of it. He had set off to Egypt in competition with Germany's greatest national rival and his own personal adversary, and he, not Pasteur, had solved the case and had shown himself the world's greatest medical detective. Koch would later say that the medal from von Bismarck was his favorite honor, since he could wear it like a military decoration.

Within a year, Koch was invited to run a new Institute of Hygiene at the University of Berlin and was given a medical professorship at the university. Virchow continued to push against Koch. "As far as we are concerned," he said, "hygiene is in the same category as forensic medicine, an applied science which has neither its own methods nor its own concepts." But he lost this argument; Koch's star now shone brighter than Virchow's. The new institute opened on July 1, 1885.

No sooner had the institute opened its doors, though, than word of a new discovery came from Paris: a new vaccine. It seemed that while Koch was in India chasing cholera, Pasteur's colleague Émile Roux had been investigating rabies, a disease more notable for the terror it caused than its overall mortality. Roux had developed what appeared to be a promising vaccine, but he had been unable to test it until a rabid dog mauled a nine-year-old boy. Throwing caution aside, Pasteur (a nondoctor) took it upon himself to administer the vaccine. It's not certain that the boy would have in fact developed the disease— the risk after such exposure is estimated at about 15 percent—but he lived, and Pasteur was hailed as a savior once again. After a few months, he had assembled further evidence for the vaccine; more than seven hundred people had been given inoculations after bites, with just one case of rabies and death. It seemed that for each of Koch's discoveries, Pasteur answered with one of his own.

Unfortunately, his new institute forced Koch to put aside his detective work and concentrate on administrative and teaching duties. His lab, by this point, had drawn some of the greatest scientists in Germany. There was Paul Ehrlich, of course, and also Emil von Behring, who began to work with Ehrlich on diphtheria. Their effort would result in the development of an antitoxin for the disease. (The work would earn von Behring the Nobel Prize in 1901.) There, too, was Kitasato Shibasaburo, the Japanese physician who came to Berlin in 1885 to study under Koch and who would later discover both the tetanus and bubonic plague bacteria. Though all this work took place under his leadership, Koch himself had little involvement in the research. He had several courses to teach, weekly lectures to give, and numerous laboratories to supervise. He established a new *Journal of Hygiene* to publish the work, but he was principally an administrator, not a researcher. "Herr Koch has nothing directly to do with our work," noted an American scientist who worked at the institute during this time. "He has just now something of more importance than the teaching of 'bugs.'"

Meanwhile, Koch's marriage was disintegrating. The relationship hadn't been particularly happy for several years, which wasn't helped by Koch's frequent absences. He began to take long vacations to Switzerland with friends, leaving Emma and daughter, Gertrud, at home. On at least one occasion, he wrote his wife that he was extending his stay for two weeks; would she please send Trudy along by herself to join him?

Surely it could have gone this way for years; a marriage gone cold was not out of the ordinary in those days when divorce was the greater sin. Except that in 1890, Koch, forty-six, met a young art student, just seventeen years old, by the name of Hedwig Freiburg. The girl seemed to spark something in Koch, a resolve to shake off his administrative yoke and return to the laboratory. Perhaps he wanted to impress young Hedwig. Perhaps he wanted to best Pasteur yet again. Whatever the reason, Koch began to spend more time in his private lab, down a long hallway from the general facilities. His colleagues had little sense of what he was doing in there, what sort of experiments he was conducting, but judging from the many dead guinea pigs coming out of the lab, they knew he was hard at work.

At long last he had returned to tuberculosis. But this time, he wasn't merely investigating questions of causality. This time he wanted glory. This time he wanted a cure.

THERE HAD, OF COURSE, BEEN MANY CURES FOR TUBERCULOSIS OVER the past decade, the past century, the past millennium. The trouble was none of them seemed to work.

In the seventeenth century the English philosopher John Locke endorsed horse riding as a genuine cure. He had seen it work firsthand, after a doctor ordered a friend to ride six or seven miles a day, until he reached 150 miles. "When he had travelled half the way," Locke reported, "his Diarrhoea stopped, and at last he came to ye end of his journey and was pretty well (at least somewhat better). . . . And in four days he came up to London perfectly cured."

In the mid-eighteenth century, before he became one of the most extreme voices of the French Revolution, Jean-Paul Marat practiced medicine in Paris, where he peddled an "antipulmonic water" for consumption. It appears to have been limewater, or calcium hydroxide, and altogether worthless, but Marat made a fortune on it. Folk cures were equally absurd. Milk from donkeys was believed to be curative, as was mutton fat. The proverbial leeches were widely used for tuberculosis, on a scale that's staggering to consider today. In France, the epicenter of bleeding in Europe, leech usage soared early in the nineteenth century, rising from 3 million leeches used in 1824–25 to a staggering 41.5 million in 1843 (a shortage in domestic leeches meant that most of these leeches were imported); a great number of these were used for tuberculars.

Some argued that playing musical instruments exposed one to the disease, while others—including Adolphe Sax, inventor of the saxophone—argued that wind instruments strengthened the lungs and were a worthy treatment. Opium was widely used and considered effective. Even a professed skeptic, the French physician Pierre Louis, did some tests and came away hopeful that it helped. "It frequently produces so material an improvement in chronic phthisis, that the patients fancy themselves cured, or almost cured, after having taken a few doses," Louis noted. Alas, though those few doses of the narcotic surely made the patient feel better, they did nothing to abate the progress of the disease.

There was also a blood remedy, in particular the blood of freshly slaughtered animals. A visitor to the Union Stock Yards in Chicago around 1890 reported that every day outside the gates there were "many regular visitors who daily drink blood, while warm from the animal, as a cure for consumption." Others believed that the blood of a species immune to tuberculosis would be a cure. In the 1880s, doctors at the Sorbonne in Paris experimented with transfusing dogs' blood into humans. (They also tried the blood of goats.) The results were promising, an American medical journal reported: "There has been neither pain, fever, reaction nor ultimate blood poisoning. . . . Appetite and sleep returned, weight increased and depression gave way to cheerfulness." What became of such research one can only speculate.

Perhaps the most popular cure was cod-liver oil. A by-product of Europe's thriving trade in codfish, cod-liver oil was seen as a cure-all for much of the nineteenth century. Its value for tuberculosis was first tested by Dr. C. J. B. Williams of the Brompton Hospital for Consumption in London. Williams swore by the stuff for more than thirty years, during which period many tons were dispensed out of his hospital. He wrote several articles attesting to its efficacy, claiming it was "more beneficial in the treatment of Pulmonary Consumption than any agent, dietetic, or regimental, that has yet been employed." This enthusiasm, inevitably, sparked a trade in rip-off oils, with many cheaper fats and greases bleached and sold as oil from cod; lard, whale blubber, and "tanner's oil" (the runoff from slaughterhouses) were common substitutes. Though cod-liver oil is now recognized as having valuable nutritional benefits, largely due to the presence of omega-3 fatty acids that may reduce risk of heart disease, as a treatment for tuberculosis, it has negligible benefits.

Ironically, the germ theory itself gave birth to the most brazen of all quack cures, the Microbe Killer, a tonic sold by the legendary American huckster William Radam. A gardener in Austin, Texas, Radam read about the growing authority of Europe's microbe hunters and was inspired to use the sheen of science to make a killing. In 1887 he began selling a potion that, he claimed, had been specifically engineered to vanquish microbes. (He was clever enough first to patent and trademark his discovery.) "It is pure water," Radam explained, "permeated with gases which are essential to the nourishment of the system, and in which micro-organisms cannot live and propagate, or fermentation exist." Boosted by an innovative nationwide advertising campaign in the United States, the Microbe Killer made Radam rich, allowing him to move from Texas to a luxury apartment overlooking

New York's Central Park. He died in 1902, but his heirs continued to sell the cure until 1912, by which time the Food and Drug Act finally empowered the government to forbid the sale of false cures. Federal agents heard news that a freight train was en route from New York to Minneapolis carrying a massive shipment of the Microbe Killer. They intercepted the train, seized the haul, and destroyed the bottles, burying the debris in a pit in St. Paul. Radam's company was soon out of business.

Some desperate souls turned to surgical treatments, and several highly experimental and potentially deadly procedures were tested in the late nineteenth century. In a thoracoplasty, a surgeon would remove several ribs from the patient, deforming the chest wall with the intention of collapsing the lungs, hoping to give the patient some relief and, perhaps, allowing the infected lung to heal. In an artificial pneumothorax, a hole was punched in the chest wall and gas (air or oxygen) injected into the lungs; the gas was intended either to kill the germs or to soothe the infected lung. In a phrenic crush, the phrenic nerve, which controls the diaphragm, would be cut, collapsing the lung, thus closing the injury. And there was the thoracotomy, the removal of a lung or a lobe of the lung. These procedures were as grisly as they sound, with high fatality rates and low rates of success. But such was the desperation of those with TB, and such was the prolonged course of the disease, that many underwent these treatments hoping for a more comfortable life on the other side of recovery.

Finally, there were the climate cures. The first sanitariums for consumptives opened in the last years of the eighteenth century, but it wasn't until 1840, when George Bodington opened a facility devoted to the treatment of consumption in Birmingham, England, that these institutions began to spread widely across Europe and the United States. Part of the argument for sanitariums was that "purer air" would invigorate weak lungs. But beyond that, the theories were contradictory. Some believed that high mountain air was most beneficial, while others advocated seaside locations, where the ocean breezes would bathe the lungs in warm air. Still others advocated dry desert conditions. Sanitariums sprang up in locations as diverse as Sante Fe, New Mexico, and Davos, Switzerland.

Inside these facilities, the treatments were as varied as the locations. While some institutions advocated vigorous exercise, the better to strengthen the lungs, others rendered their patients completely immobile. This meant more than mere bed rest. Patients were required to lie prone in their beds twenty-four hours a day, with orders not to stir. Nurses would spoon food into patients' mouths and bring them bedpans for relief. This could go on for many months or as long as a year. Needless to say, such conditions were miserable and debilitating for patients—psyches were scarred, careers abandoned, marriages ruined, families lost. It makes one wonder how accurate was the inscription on the largest hotel in Davos, *Hilares mox sani*, "The merry are soon cured."

This steady parade of overhyped cures speaks to the desperation of the sufferers. With each new treatment, hope was refueled and then disappointed. So on to the next. The market was always ready to offer something new.

If it was torment for patients, it was bleak for physicians as well. As a doctor from Mansfield, Ohio, lamented in 1890:

We have tried in vain for centuries to "cure" consumption. People by the thousand and hundreds of thousands have flocked from one health resort to another, vainly seeking to free themselves from the lion grip of pulmonary consumption; they have, figuratively speaking, soaked themselves in cod liver oil, and clad themselves, inside and out, with iron; they have loaded their poor stomachs with the hypophosphites, and been pumped with the pneumatic cabinet, and injected with carbonic acid gas; but the end was all the same—it was only a question of time until the funeral knell sounded the requiem of their departed spirits.

Harvard anatomist and author Oliver Wendell Holmes in 1860 wrote off altogether the effort of curing the disease. "I firmly believe that if the whole materia medica, *as now used,* could be sunk to the bottom of the sea, it would be all the better for mankind—and all the worse for the fishes."

From today's vantage point, some of these cures look ridiculous or barbaric. Medical and surgical treatments are available now for a broad range of diseases—diabetes, heart disease, HIV/AIDS, glaucoma, certain cancers, tetanus, strep and staph infections, and pneumonia— so we assume that scientists, somewhere, are going down a checklist, ticking off diseases one by one.

This was the premise, after all, of America's first "war on cancer," declared by President Richard Nixon in 1971. The expectation then was that science, having been called to war, would take five years to find the cure. But in the more than four decades since then, many of today's cancer patients have scarcely a better chance of survival than they would have faced forty years ago. Yet the conversation around cancer continues to invoke the word *cure,* and the term is nearly as common when discussing other chronic or life-threatening ailments. We are too easily beguiled into thinking that a great remedy is around the next bend, that every disease can be cured. The danger lies where, in our desperation, we fail to distinguish between the true break-through and the sham cure.

BY THE SUMMER OF 1890, KOCH BELIEVED HE WAS ONTO SOME-thing. He was searching for some internal antiseptic, a chemical that might be ingested or injected and rid the body of the tuberculosis bac-terium from within. Using those hordes of guinea pigs, he worked his way through a long list of possible agents: acids, alkalis, toxins, and dyes. None of them panned out. Then he tried a new substance, a lymph, which seemed to have some sort of reaction in animals. In

Koch's experiments, guinea pigs that had been infected with tub
losis tended to live between six and eight weeks. But those inocul,
with this new substance—he would call it tuberculin—lived longer.
Most curiously, treated tissue had necrotized, or died—it "rather
melts or wastes away," as Koch wrote in his notebook. This wasn't the
expected result: Rather than treating the infection, as an antiseptic
would, the substance seemed to kill off the flesh that the microbes fed
upon. Though unexpected, it seemed a promising effect. Indeed, it
tracked with Koch's success elsewhere.

The effect is known as amplification, an increase from one state to
another. Amplification had been the essential tool in Koch's cabinet,
the phenomenon common to so much of his work. Microscopy is
amplification: boosting the perceived size of an object from the invisible to the visible. And cultures work by amplification, deliberately
growing a small number of bacteria into a much larger quantity. In
these cases, amplification was a pragmatic tool; it made microbes
visible. (Amplification is still an essential principle of laboratory
science today. The traditional technique for sequencing DNA involves
amplifying one piece of DNA into billions, making it easier to read
the sequence of nucleotides and thus diagnose disease or genetic conditions.)

So when Koch saw something like amplification after treatment
with tuberculin, he was encouraged. By killing off the underlying
flesh, tuberculin seemed to undermine the parasitic strategy of the
bacteria, giving them no place to roost. Today we understand this sort
of thinking as confirmation bias. Koch wanted to believe his treatment
was working, so he looked for evidence that it was. And the necrotized flesh gave Koch an explanation for how tuberculin worked. Unfortunately, he failed to apply his own microscopic techniques and
wait to see if the bacteria had been truly vanquished.

By June, Koch decided that he was satisfied with his animal
experiments. It was time to test the substance on healthy human

subjects—starting with himself and his teenage mistress. He took a syringe, filled it with two or three milliliters of the fluid, and injected it into his arm. Later he repeated the procedure on Hedwig. Two assistants were next, and in each case the reaction was similar: "3 to 4 hours after the injection: aching limbs, fatigue, tendency to cough, rapidly increasing breathing difficulties," he wrote in his notebook; "in the 5th hour unusually violent shivering set in, lasting for about an hour. At the same time there was nausea and vomiting as the body temperature rose to 39.6 centigrade; after about 12 hours all these complaints receded."

Today we recognize this as an immune reaction, a concept that was then only just emerging (advanced by scientists working in Koch's own laboratory). The spike in temperature—normal human temperature is thirty-seven degrees centigrade—was especially exciting to Koch, as it seemed to be another manifestation of amplification, evoking a "fever cure," the ancient notion that a fever burns disease out of the body. (At the time, fever cure was still a popular idea. It faded with the development of aspirin and other pain relievers at the turn of the twentieth century, but it is finding new traction today; recent research has shown little to no benefit to reducing a fever through aspirin or other anti-inflammatories, while there may be potential benefits to letting a fever run its course.) But to the extent that it echoed folk wisdom rather than evidence-based science, the appearance of fever should have provoked caution in Koch. In fact, it contradicted one of his favorite dictums, that "the least reliable results were obtained from experiences gathered at the sickbed." But Koch was impatient for success. He had let his biases get the better of him.

ON AUGUST 3, 1890, THE TENTH INTERNATIONAL MEDICAL CONgress opened in Berlin. Some six thousand physicians and scientists had come to Berlin, filling the Circus Renz, a massive circular building in central Berlin. The space was turned out splendidly, with a triumphal arch of evergreen festooned with flowers and flags from all nations. This Tenth Congress was the successor to the London congress where, nine years earlier, Pasteur had reported on his anthrax vaccine and where Koch had demonstrated his meticulous laboratory techniques. This time the audience hoped for even more miracles.

It was an oppressively hot day. Outside, the air was muggy and thick; inside, it was downright suffocating, with the thousands of attendees pressed together and hundreds of gas and electric lights radiating heat. On the main platform, a colossal statue of Asclepius, the Greek god of medicine and healing, stood guard over the proceedings, holding a snake and a staff.

With a dozen German dignitaries and ministers at his side, Rudolf Virchow, the congress president, rose to call the meeting to order. He was greeted by cheers and applause. "In this imperfect world all practical progress is made only step by step," Virchow said, making sure to note the accomplishments of German science, in particular Berlin's new sanitation system, which he had championed personally. Next, Joseph Lister offered an update on his antiseptic techniques. (He was done with carbolic acid, he explained, and now preferred a salt of cyanide of mercury and zinc, or a dilution of mercuric chloride.)

Then came Koch, who began by offering broad observations on the state of bacteriological research. The size of the hall and the lack of amplification made for horrible acoustics, and the audience struggled to make sense of what Koch was saying. He continued for several minutes, until he turned to the one question that, he said, was often asked of him: "What has been achieved by all the arduous labor that has been invested in the examination of bacteria?" He recognized the validity of the question and wanted to highlight the practical benefits. "There must be a remedy for tuberculosis," he said, explaining how he'd been testing all sorts of substances for their curative properties on the disease: ethereal oils, naphthylamine, paratoluidin, xylidine, tar dyes, mercury, and silver and gold compounds. "All of these substances," he reported, "remained absolutely without effect if tried on tuberculous animals."

Then Koch hinted at something new. "I have at last hit upon a substance which has the power of preventing the growth of tubercle bacilli, not only in a test tube, but in the body of an animal." Noting that his experiments were ongoing and not yet definitive, he could only hint at their implications.

> All I can say at present is that if guinea pigs are treated they cannot be inoculated with tuberculosis, and guinea pigs which already are in the late stages of the disease are completely cured, although the body suffers no ill effects from the treatment. From these experiments, I will draw no other conclusion at present than that it is possible to render pathogenic bacteria within the body harmless without ill effect on the body itself.

Koch teased, but volunteered no specifics, no details on what his substance might be. Indeed, he was so restrained that, in the days after the congress, the reports of his remarks were generally tepid. "Dr. Koch was shrewd enough not to name his 'cure,' so we did not learn much from the distinguished director," an American physician reported. *The Lancet* was even more dubious. "Dr. Koch's address treated chiefly of what is already known. The new points were . . . some observations on tuberculosis . . . and on the possible curative treatment of phthisis." Nonetheless, the idea was now out there—there should be a real cure, and he might have it.

Why would the invariably discreet scientist take such a risk? To some extent, he was doing his part as a good German. *The Lancet* hinted at such. The German government, keenly aware that the world would be attending the Belin congress, apparently wanted some show of prowess from its scientists. The politicians had pushed on the host committee, and the committee had turned to Koch, imploring him to reveal some great progress from his laboratory. The journal later reported:

> Koch, like all scientific men, has his own methods of working, and his own system of declaring his results. He had never yet rushed into print with a discovery until he has been sure of his facts, and all who are in any way acquainted with the circumstances under which Koch was practically compelled by his Government superiors and by his colleagues to make the premature statement at the International Medical Congress in Berlin will sympathise most deeply with him that he was compelled to break through his usual reticence.

Regardless, now that the word was out about his work, Koch spent the next weeks in a fervor. He delegated his administrative and teaching duties at the Institute of Hygiene and turned to the experiments full-time. First on his agenda was to test tuberculin on human subjects—not just to test the safety of the substance on healthy subjects, as he had on himself and his young friend, but to administer actual therapeutic doses to consumptives. By September, those experiments were under way at Berlin's Charité hospital, with several patients receiving regular injections of tuberculin, under the supervision of Dr. Ernst von Bergmann, an esteemed surgeon at the University of Berlin.

In October, word of these human experiments began to spread. In a brief update on November 1, *The Lancet* advised that doctors and the public itself heed Koch's trademark caution. "Indeed, apart from the fact that we may be on the verge of a revolution in therapeutics, it may be said that bacteriology itself is on its trial in this momentous investigation."

By mid-November, Koch was ready to reveal something more. On November 13, in Berlin's *Deutsche Medizinische Wochenschrift,* he published "A Further Communication on a Remedy for Tuberculosis." (This report was quickly translated and published across the world; Conan Doyle read it in the *BMJ* two days later.) Up front, Koch acknowledged that his research was not yet complete.

> It was originally my intention to complete the research . . . before publishing anything on the subject. But, in spite of all precautions, too many accounts have reached the public, and those in an exaggerated and distorted form, so that it seems imperative, in order to prevent all false impressions, to give at once a review of the position of the subject at the present stage of inquiry.

The caveats, though, soon gave way to the explicit suggestion that he'd made a stunning discovery. His substance appeared to have a dramatic effect on tubercular tissue, he explained, a reaction that was both pronounced and almost certainly therapeutic. Repeatedly he used one word to describe this new substance: *Heilmittel,* he called it. "The remedy."

How much would "Koch's lymph," as tuberculin began to be called, cost? How much was available?

Koch was coy on all counts. He described his remedy only as "a brownish transparent liquid" and failed to elaborate. "As regards the origin and the preparation of the remedy I am unable to make any statement, as my research is not yet concluded; I reserve this for a future communication." As to where and when his remedy might be available, his paper did offer a suggestion:

Doctors wishing to make investigations with the remedy at present, can obtain it from Dr. A. Libbertz, Luneburger Strasse, 28, Berlin, N. W., who has undertaken the preparation of the remedy, with my own and Dr. Pfuhl's cooperation. But I must remark that the quantity prepared at present is but small, and that larger quantities will not be obtainable for some weeks.

That supply, though, was soon exhausted, and tuberculin would quickly become perhaps the most sought-after substance in the world.

As Koch described it, tuberculin worked by provoking an intense reaction in the tissue and metabolism of consumptive patients. The response typically began with a strong fever, shaking, and general malaise. Infected tissue swelled up quickly, with noticeable reddening on scrofular wounds in the skin. Gradually, the infected flesh began to die. Koch noted that "the way which this process works is not yet fully understood because histological analyses are still not available. But one issue is already clear: the material does not kill the bacilli in the tissue directly, but instead, the tissue containing tubercle bacilli is affected by this treatment."

Curiously, Koch provided little in the way of actual statistical evidence to substantiate his claims. He justified this omission as one of professional courtesy:

I have purposely omitted statistical accounts and descriptions of individual cases, because the medical men who furnished us with patients for our investigation have themselves decided to publish the description of their cases, and I wished my account to be as objective as possible, leaving to them all that is purely personal.

Data or no data, Koch's news was immediately hailed worldwide as the long-awaited cure for tuberculosis. "He has given the world a

safe means with which to combat the angel of death named Consumption," wrote the *Vossische Zeitung*, one of Germany's leading
newspapers, "for if that dreadful illness is recognized in time and
treated properly, it is curable." In America, a special cable dispatch of
The Medical News described it as "the seed of a discovery the extent of
whose fruit cannot be grasped by the human mind, and which bids
fair to surpass the triumph of Jenner in his warfare against smallpox."
On November 16 the front page of *The New York Times* declared the
news with the headline "KOCH'S GREAT TRIUMPH," hailing
the discovery "as one greater than Jenner's." Some desperate souls
bought rail tickets to Berlin in the hope of convincing Koch to add
them to his experiments.

There was an immediate demand for additional information and
for a demonstration of the therapy. This was hastily arranged for November 17, in Berlin. Von Bergmann would present evidence on his
trials; Koch himself would be in attendance. With barely a few hours'
notice, physicians and scientists from throughout Europe hastily re-
arranged their schedules in order to be in Berlin. Soon, Berlin's hotels
and lodgings were filled with more than a thousand physicians—
among them Arthur Conan Doyle.

CONAN DOYLE ARRIVED IN BERLIN ON SUNDAY, NOVEMBER 16. HE
was exhausted from his travels but invigorated. On the train, he'd met
Malcolm Morris, a successful London dermatologist also en route to
the demonstration. Morris was accompanied by a patient with lupus,
and he had some hope of getting his patient enrolled in Koch's
remedy. They fell to talking, and Morris, who was twelve years older,
saw something of himself in the younger doctor. Both were from
Catholic families, and both had begun as general practitioners in the
provinces. But Morris had aimed higher and broken out, and he urged
Conan Doyle to do the same. "He assured me that I was wasting my
life in the provinces and had too small a field for my activities. He

insisted that I should leave general practice and go to London," Conan Doyle said later. Morris suggested that he choose some specialty—the eye, Conan Doyle answered. Just right, Morris thought, suggesting, "thus, you will have a nice clean life with plenty of leisure for your literature."

This, of course, was the path that Conan Doyle had proposed for himself the previous year, when he allowed himself to dream that *Micah Clarke* might be a bestseller. But having that plan endorsed by Morris was something different.

Conan Doyle had been an admirer of the germ theory since his medical school days; as he demonstrated in his "Life and Death in the Blood" essay, he recognized the power of both Koch's and Pasteur's work. But of the two, it was Koch with whom he was more philosophically aligned. Pasteur was an impetuous scientist, quick with a hypothesis even when he lacked evidence to support it. Sometimes, as in the case of silkworms, this could set him back years and cost dearly those who believed his conclusions. Moreover, Pasteur was a chemist by training, not a physician like Conan Doyle.

Koch, on the other hand, was a physician, and he had risen from obscurity, just as Conan Doyle yearned to. Koch had made his name by assembling evidence first; he built his case slowly and deliberately, just as Dr. Joseph Bell had taught Conan Doyle to do. In Berlin, Conan Doyle would finally have the opportunity to witness this process firsthand.

When his train arrived in Berlin, Conan Doyle headed straight to the British embassy, where he hoped to get the ambassador's help in securing one last seat for the next day's demonstration. Alas, he went away empty-handed; tickets were "simply not to be had and neither money nor interest could procure them." Not to be dissuaded, Conan Doyle found Robert Koch's home. If he couldn't get in by official sanction, perhaps he could impress the great scientist himself that he was worthy of a seat. Conan Doyle knocked on the door and waited.

A butler answered, and Conan Doyle, who had learned German

during his year in Austria, explained why he was there. The butler invited Conan Doyle to step inside and wait while he went upstairs to tell Herr Koch who was at the door.

Scarcely twenty-four hours before, Conan Doyle had been at home in Southsea, and now here he was in Berlin, in Koch's own house. Not only might he find his way into the demonstration, but he was about to meet the man whose work he had followed so closely for the past decade. Perhaps his exhausting trip would all be worth it.

As he waited for the butler to return, the postman arrived to deliver the day's mail. He carried a large sack and emptied its contents upon a desk in the foyer. A cascade of letters tumbled out, spilling over the tabletop and onto the floor. Conan Doyle sneaked a look at the pile and saw postmarks from all over the world. He realized that these envelopes were likely pleas from a thousand consumptives. These letters, Conan Doyle said later, were pieces of "all the sad broken lives and wearied hearts which were turning in hope to Berlin."

The butler returned and gave him the disappointing news: Herr Koch was unavailable. He would not see the unknown English visitor. Crushed, Conan Doyle thanked the butler and walked out. As Conan Doyle noted soon after, "to the Englishman in Berlin, and indeed to the German also, it is at present very much easier to see the bacillus of Koch than to catch even the most fleeting glimpse of its discoverer."

Conan Doyle found lodging for the night and, the next morning, headed straight to the lecture hall at the university. He passed a few deutsche marks to a porter guarding a door and slipped inside the outer hall. At an inner door, to the hall itself, he again offered a porter a few marks to let him through, but this one took offense, and Conan Doyle was rudely dismissed. People with tickets began to crowd through the door, bustling past Conan Doyle. He halfheartedly tried to blend in among them and slip through in the throng, but the porter called him out and pushed him back with a scold. Conan Doyle could do nothing but stand there.

At last, the lecture hall was full, and Dr. von Bergmann came to the door with a few assistants, ready to begin the demonstration. Conan Doyle had one last chance. Begging von Bergmann's pardon, he stopped him and asked for a seat. "I have come a thousand miles," he implored. "May I not come in?" In ninety-nine cases out of a hundred, Conan Doyle figured, the request would have worked.

But von Bergmann was the hundredth man. "There's no place," the German answered. "Perhaps you would like to take my place? That is the only place left. Yes, yes, take my place, by all means. My classes are filled with Englishmen already." Von Bergmann's coterie laughed at his mean joke, and Conan Doyle backed away.

Conan Doyle turned toward the door in defeat, but just then another man stopped him. "See here," he said to Conan Doyle. "That was bad behavior." It was Henry Hartz, an American doctor from Detroit. He was headed into the hall and had heard von Bergmann's snide insult. Quickly, Conan Doyle explained his predicament. Hartz couldn't give up his ticket, but he offered to meet Conan Doyle that afternoon and share his notes from the lecture. Conan Doyle readily agreed. His trip might be saved after all.

That afternoon, he met Hartz and read the notes closely, making his own copy. The two physicians got on well enough that Hartz invited Conan Doyle to join him the next morning on a visit to von Bergmann's ward, to see firsthand the patients being treated with tuberculin.

That next morning, the seventeenth of November, Conan Doyle and Hartz visited von Bergmann's clinic. Conan Doyle was taken aback by what he saw. "A long and grim array they were of twisted joints, rotting bones, and foul ulcers of the skin, all more or less under the benign influence of the inoculation," Conan Doyle described. "Here and there I saw a patient, bright-eyed, flushed, and breathing heavily, who was in the stage of reaction after the administration of the injection; for it cannot be too clearly understood that the first effect of the virus [the remedy] is to intensify the symptoms, to raise the temperature to an almost dangerous degree, and in every way to make the patient worse instead of better." He then visited two other clinics where tuberculin was being tested on human subjects, and at last found his way inside Koch's own laboratory on Klosterstrasse.

There he was again denied an audience with Koch, but he did get a glimpse of what was one of the world's greatest medical laboratories. "It is a large square chamber," Conan Doyle described it, "well lit and lofty, with rows of microscopes bristling along the deal tables which line it upon every side. Bunsen burners, reservoirs of distilled water, freezing machines for the cutting of microscopic sections, and every other conceivable aid to the bacteriological student, lie ready to his hand." He noted the array of samples laid out neatly on the tables, potatoes smudged with colonies of red or blue or black molds and fungi. And he got a chance to look under a microscope, one that Koch himself perhaps looked under, to see the spores and dots of *Mycobacterium tuberculosis*, *Vibrio cholerae*, and *Bacillus anthracis*. They looked so insignificant to him, barely more than grains of pepper, yet thanks to Koch, there was no doubt of their great and terrifying power. Conan Doyle noted the paradox:

> It is a strange thing to look upon these utterly insignificant creatures, and to realize that in one year they would claim more victims from the human race than all the tigers who have ever trod a jungle. A satire, indeed, it is upon the majesty of man when we look at these infinitesimal and contemptible creatures which have it in their power to overthrow the strongest intellect and to shatter the most robust frame.

THAT AFTERNOON, CONAN DOYLE RETURNED TO HIS HOTEL ROOM and began writing his first dispatch, a letter to *The Daily Telegraph*. Though the editors titled the letter "The Consumption Cure," Conan Doyle's frank assessment was that it almost certainly was nothing of the sort. "Great as is Koch's discovery, there can be no question that our knowledge of it is still very incomplete, and that it leaves large issues open to question," he wrote. "The sooner that this is recognised the less chance will there be of serious disappointment among those who are looking to Berlin for a panacea for their own or their friends' ill-health."

He described the rounds he'd taken in the Berlin clinics, noting that Koch himself couldn't claim that his substance actually killed bacteria. Conan Doyle suggested a sobering analogy: "It is as if a man whose house was infested with rats were to remove the marks of the creatures every morning and expect in that way to get rid of them." This was clearly no cure, at least in Dr. Conan Doyle's assessment.

With that, Conan Doyle headed back to Southsea, where he had a few days to craft his essay for *The Review of Reviews*. The essay was a much more deeply considered exploration of Koch and his work than the *Telegraph* letter, four thousand words in all. It described the man down to his "small, grey, and searching" eyes and "slightly retroussé nose." Conan Doyle covered Koch's years in Göttingen working with Jacob Henle and captured his years of obscurity in Wöllstein: "Poor, humble, unknown, isolated from sympathy and from the scientific appliances which are the necessary tools of the investigator." It's a vivid portrait, and remarkably spot-on, as if Conan Doyle had been somehow observing Koch during those years. In a way, perhaps, he was, since the words could equally describe Conan Doyle: "He was a man of too strong a character to allow himself to be warped by the position in which he found himself, or to be diverted from the line of work which was most congenial to his nature."

Conan Doyle succinctly summarized Koch's work on anthrax and cholera, crediting his research on wound infections as vindicating Lister's efforts. He praised Koch as the "great master mind" and the "noblest German of them all." But ultimately, Conan Doyle came to the same, cold assessment that he had in *The Daily Telegraph*: Koch's lymph almost certainly had no effect in actually treating the disease. "Unfortunately, it is evident that the system soon establishes a tolerance to the injected fluid, so that the time must apparently come when the continually renewed tubercle tissue will refuse to respond to the remedy. In the case of true phthisis of the lungs . . . the evidence is so slight that we can only regard it as an indication and a hope, rather than a proof."

The remedy might not be altogether useless, though. Conan Doyle suggested that it likely had great value as a diagnostic for tuberculosis, in a smaller dose (which, as it happened, would turn out to be exactly its true utility). He concludes by noting Koch's own candor and thoroughness; he fully expected Koch to emerge from his isolation and volunteer "the weak points and flaws in his own system."

Back in Berlin, though, Koch was busy contending with the frenzy that he'd set off: the experiments, the ravenous appetite for tuberculin, the requests from press and politicians and the public. We can't say whether he was aware of Conan Doyle's critical assessment; even had he been, he would likely have dismissed it as ill-informed speculation, more noise from the cynical mob. Nonetheless, amid the hysteria breaking out throughout Europe over Koch's remedy, Conan Doyle's was almost certainly the first thorough appraisal of tuberculin, based on an examination of patients under treatment. It was a rigorous debunking, using Koch's own model of logic and analysis to reveal his remedy's weaknesses.

The only question was, which of the two men would the world believe?

PART III

CHAPTER 8

1891 · The Fall of Dr. Koch

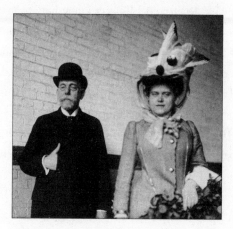

Robert Koch and his second wife, Hedwig, in 1908

All across Berlin, the letters began to pile up. Koch's announcement of his remedy had directed doctors who wished to make their own investigations to his colleague Dr. Libbertz. And so, every day, the postman would arrive at Libbertz's office and drop a knee-high pile of letters upon the floor, each message a plea for some small amount of the remedy. When word got out that the Berlin clinic of Dr. Georg Cornet had some stock, the letters arrived there as well. "There was no stopping [them]," Cornet observed. "Like a growing avalanche, letters and telegrams from all countries and in every language reached Koch and were passed on to me, and within a few days my correspondence also numbered in the hundreds."

The appeals came from physicians hoping to secure some lymph for their patients; from hospitals and sanitariums hoping to provide some last treatment in their wards; and mostly, from the patients who had been struck by the disease. They were all desperate for what might be the only chance for survival.

Actual doses of the remedy, meanwhile, were scarce, almost mythic. The production process was slow, and since the substance was a secret, only Drs. Koch and Libbertz knew how to manufacture it. Libbertz's supplies were soon gone, and he expected it would be months before there was enough supply again to meet the demand.

But that demand was unquenchable—it comprised, after all, a quarter of all humanity or more. These were millions of people who had little hope, until Koch had offered a bit more. So they sent letters, hoping that theirs might land somewhere and earn enough notice, enough sympathy, to merit a dose of Koch's remedy. Their stories were both uniquely and uniformly tragic. Charles Pratt lived in Minneapolis, Minnesota, when his daughter developed TB. In search of a cure, the family subsequently sold their home and moved to consumptive colonies in Phoenix, then Tucson, their savings dwindling with each passing day. By the time word of Koch's cure reached the western United States, the Pratt family was living in a tent in Idaho at 3,500 feet. But the disease wouldn't release its grasp on the girl. "Is there any place in the world where the Koch method of treatment by inoculation is so successfully tried, as to make it worthwhile to go there?" the desperate father wrote to a Philadelphia physician who he had heard was influential. "Pardon this from a stranger."

From Paris, Pasteur sent a telegram congratulating Koch for his efforts. Even the French press joined in the acclaim: "All the world rejoices in the humanitarian significance of Koch's discovery," one Paris reporter offered. In the meantime, Koch dispatched his assistants throughout Europe to conduct public demonstrations of the remedy, including in London, Edinburgh, and Paris.

The acclaim, though, was tempered by concerns that Koch had been uncharacteristically secretive about his remedy. He, of all people, should be keen to divulge it, in the interest of science. After all, as *The Review of Reviews* noted in an introduction to Conan Doyle's essay, "according to the rule of the profession, no cures wrought by secret remedies can ever be examined into. All dealers in secret remedies are quacks. But Dr. Koch, as far as the retention of the secret of his remedy goes, is as much a quack as Sequah or Count Mattei." Sequah and Count Mattei were the two most notorious quacks of the day, and ordinarily they would be held up as Koch's opposite. Clearly, his reputation was on the line: What, exactly, was in this lymph? Why, people wanted to know, was this a *secret* remedy? Why wouldn't he share his discovery with the world, as he had every time before? What was Koch afraid of?

Today, the gold standard for medical research is the randomized clinical trial, or RCT. A group of patients, all suffering from a condition, are randomly divided into two groups: One is the case group, which will receive the treatment (typically a drug), and the other is the control group, which will receive a benign placebo (typically a sugar pill). The experiment must be double-blind, meaning neither the patient nor the investigators know which patients are receiving which treatment. (The results are monitored by a lab assistant, not the principal investigators.) In this way, wishful thinking on the part of both the study subjects and the researchers is minimized.

The basic structure for a clinical trial dates back to British naval surgeon James Lind, who wanted to examine whether citrus fruits helped sailors avoid scurvy, the nasty wasting away of connective tissue caused by a deficiency of vitamin C. Though lemons and limes had occasionally been thought effective against the disease, that knowledge was anecdotal. In 1747, Lind set about to test the theory rigorously. He divided twelve scurvy-afflicted sailors into six groups of two. He gave them the same diet, but each pair received a different supplement: cider, sulfuric acid, vinegar, seawater, barley water, or oranges and lemons. After less than a week, the duo getting the fruit had recovered, while the others were still suffering. Lind published his results in 1753, though it would take fifty years (and the deaths of thousands more sailors) before his results were put into practice.

The experimental method got another boost in the 1830s, when French physician Pierre Louis took the then-radical position of urging his colleagues to forsake their subjective assessments and instead apply statistical rigor to their experiments. "Let those who engage hereafter in the study of therapeutics . . . demonstrate, rigorously, the . . . degree of influence of any therapeutic agent on the duration, progress, and termination of a particular disease." (Louis would mentor Oliver Wendell Holmes when he studied in Paris.)

Despite these pioneers, the standard protocols for the RCT were developed surprisingly recently, in the 1940s and '50s, by the British epidemiologists Arthur Bradford Hill and his colleague Archie Cochrane. Cochrane's passion for the RCT is legendary: "Randomize, always randomize!" he would implore his students in Cardiff, where he taught at the Welsh National School of Medicine. Cochrane, who developed his methods as a German prisoner of war in the 1940s, was certain that if investigators knew which groups were getting which treatment, bias would inevitably slip into the analysis and destroy the credibility of an experiment. The magic of randomization is that it greatly reduces methodological biases, and it makes room for statistics. Statistical analysis is the lifeblood of contemporary science. It provides the foundation for evaluating the validity of an experiment's results and a common language for other scientists to pursue their own analogous experiments.

Study design is just one of the formalities we now take for granted in modern medical research. The second is experimental oversight, specifically an ethical review to assess whether the research itself is within the bounds of accepted values. Today, every experiment involving human subjects must be approved and monitored by an institutional review board, or IRB, an independent ethical committee

with a mandate to ensure that all human subjects are bo[...]
of possible risks and protected from any physical or [...]
harm. In the United States, IRBs are run in close affiliatio[...]
major research institutions; IRBs are also regulated by the Food and
Drug Administration.

None of this existed in Koch's day. The experiments involving tuberculin were, by today's standards, reckless, disorganized, and conducted with scant regard for individual human life. Shipments of
tuberculin were sent all over Europe, their destinations determined as
much by personal connections as by need or scientific bona fides.
Within weeks of the November demonstration, tuberculin experiments were under way in several academic clinics in Berlin and around
Europe, and in private clinics and sanatoriums around Europe and
the United States. Those with enough resources procured their own
supplies, and soon private individuals were conducting their own reg-
imens. Koch appears to have personally selected some physicians to
receive a supply of tuberculin, enough for a demonstration of its
potency, but not enough to conduct a thorough assessment of its efficacy. These experiments were more spectacle than science, and some
physicians began criticizing the whole thing as so much sensation-
alism. An anonymous letter to *The Lancet* made the point:

> Day after day the gaping multitude were informed how Dr.
> This and Dr. That, having received a sample of the precious
> fluid, had proceeded to inject it in the presence of a circle of
> admiring and envious confreres. The ceremonial, which
> might have been the performance of a sacred rite rather than
> the administration in minimal doses of hypodermic injec-
> tions of a secret remedy was ... chronicled with as much
> detail as a fashionable wedding or a public funeral.

Even when there was enough supply to afford a true experiment,
there was no such thing as a standard protocol. Each facility followed

its own interpretation of Koch's rather imprecise descriptions of proper dilution and dosage. In practice, dosages varied widely, as did the frequency and timing of injections; physicians seemed to be calibrating these factors by gut instinct, depending on the severity of a patient's symptoms. Some gave patients a course of six doses of seven milligrams each; others gave more than twenty doses of twenty or more milligrams each. Even how to administer the dose varied; Koch suggested an injection in the back, between the scapulae, but others tried injections in the arms and legs. Record keeping was haphazard at best, with most clinics noting how symptoms progressed hour by hour, but with descriptions and terminology at the discretion of the note taker. (The patient's name, age, and occupation were routinely disclosed in full, while the physician was identified only by his initials.) In some hospitals, the injections were performed almost ceremoniously. When a shipment of the remedy arrived at a hospital in Greifswald, a town on Germany's north coast, for instance, the whole staff turned out for the occasion. "Against a background of laurel bushes, doctors, nurses and patients in snowy-white garments and the chief in his black cutaway were lined up: Address by the internist, injections for a chosen group of patients, thundering hurrahs for Robert Koch."

In terms of patient response, the reactions varied widely. Some people seemed to improve almost instantaneously, such as a woman suffering from tuberculosis in her throat. After three injections, she appeared entirely cured. Others seemed only to get worse from the moment of the initial reaction, their temperature spiking and their experiencing frequent nausea and vomiting. Injections were given to patients almost randomly, for various reasons: to severely consumptive patients near death, to test the degree of their fevers; and to those suffering from nonconsumptive diseases as well, such as syphilis or meningitis, just to see how they reacted. The remedy was given to men and women; to children of eleven, six, and two and a half years old; and even to newborns, despite von Bergmann's declaration that he "considered the use of Koch's medication in children under the age of 10 extremely dangerous."

Inevitably, patients began to die in the throes of fever, their limbs thrashing violently, in what would today be recognized as shock. Worryingly, this sometimes happened even to patients whose phthisis had seemed to be in remission. Undoubtedly, some died because the general rule was to increase the dose gradually, even if low doses provoked severe reactions. In the thrall surrounding the treatment, though, these unfortunates were quickly dismissed as having been beyond help to begin with.

In all, it was an uncontrolled, absolutely chaotic process, closer to anarchy than experimentation. But the enthusiasm for a cure was such that a sense of euphoria overtook even those who should have been immune, including Lord Lister. In late 1890 he visited Berlin with his niece, who had a case of consumption. Though Koch greatly admired Lister, it would be a week before he could see him and arrange for treatment. Upon his return to London, in an address at King's College Hospital, Lister gave the remedy his full endorsement. "The effects . . . are simply astounding," he said, comparing the effect to Pasteur's anthrax vaccine. Lister even endorsed the secrecy of the cure. Even now, weeks into an experiment being conducted upon thousands of individuals across the globe, nobody outside Koch's lab knew what was being injected into so many people. "By publishing now the precise mode of preparing this material, he might do immense harm instead of good," Lister suggested. Whatever it might be, Koch's secret remedy seemed to be the cure that so many had yearned for.

ON NOVEMBER 22 (THE SAME DAY CONAN DOYLE'S PIECE APPEARED in *The Review of Reviews*), the German emperor bestowed upon Koch the Grand Cross of the Order of the Red Eagle, the government's highest decoration, typically reserved for military heroes or royalty. In part this was payback. A few months earlier, the emperor had urged Koch's patron, Minister Heinrich von Gossler, to have something spectacular on tap for the International Medical Congress that took place in Berlin in August; von Gossler had asked Koch to deliver something appropriate. He had clearly exceeded expectations.

As he watched Pasteur gain acclaim and honor in France, Koch had expected the same of his country. On October 31, when the human experiments were still in their early stages but before he had publicly disclosed the research, Koch made a formal request: He wanted a new institute dedicated to the production and study of tuberculin, with himself as its director.

He was keenly aware of the prospect of financial gain from his discovery. In his proposal, he suggested that, for six years, he be the sole beneficiary of tuberculin sales; the rights would thereafter be transferred to the German government. The money involved was not trifling: At a daily production of five hundred doses, a conservative estimate, Koch calculated that his new institute would earn 4.5 million marks a year on tuberculin. Thanks to the constant supply of people with tuberculosis, he noted, there would be a guaranteed long-term demand.

In early November, Koch and German officials reached an agreement: Koch would run an institute with two purposes: first, for clinical testing of tuberculin, and second, as a laboratory for medical research. He would get his monopoly.

No official announcement was made, but rumors soon began to spread. A London paper reported that Gerson von Bleichröder, von Bismarck's private banker, had agreed to contribute one million marks for Koch's new clinic; this was reputed to be matched by another million from the German government. Others began to speculate how much Koch would be personally profiting from the remedy. By December, his institute deal had become an outright controversy, verging on scandal. With the remedy itself still unproven, the German chancellor exercised his privilege to veto the deal, explaining it would be unseemly for Koch to be perceived as exploiting his remedy for personal gain. The negotiations were put on hold until "public opinion has a clearer idea as to the value of the medication."

Koch's continued secrecy about the actual composition of the therapy was particularly vexing. In a rare interview with the press, he offered the reason for his secrecy. He was concerned, he said, that if he disclosed the formula before his testing was complete,

> thousands of medical men, from Moscow to Buenos Aires, would tomorrow be engaged in concocting it, and injecting it for that matter. Is it far-fetched, then, for me to suppose, as I do, that more than half of these gentlemen are incompetent . . . ? Then these experiments might cause incalculable harm to thousands of innocent patients, and at the same time bring into discredit a system of treatment which, I believe, will prove a boon to mankind.

But physicians were growing suspicious. Koch's reputation had protected him so far, but as the experiments continued and expanded, more medical men began to openly voice their concerns. A Berlin colleague of Koch's, Ernst von Leyden, noted in late November that "the clinician finds himself in a peculiar position. We have received from the hands of a scientist of genius a medication for our use, yet we have no information about its nature; save for some vague conjectures, it is shrouded in mystery." In December, a doctor from Heidelberg wrote of "the unease that creeps up on every physician when he has to operate with a secret nostrum." Indeed, it's a remarkable testimony to Koch's reputation that so many physicians injected it into their patients, and that so many people from around the world continued to flock for a dose of his treatment, without the least sort of understanding of what it might be.

By year's end, the data had started to come in. It did not look good for Koch. At least sixty-nine scientific papers appeared on tuberculin, mostly case studies. The Prussian government gathered the evidence into a summary report. In these, some 2,172 people had been injected with tuberculin, receiving a total of 17,500 doses. These patients suffered from every manifestation of the disease, from pulmonary phthisis to lupus and scrofula. The results were ambiguous at best: Of 242 patients with pulmonary TB treated with tuberculin, 9 appeared to have been cured, and 131 seemed improved. Of 444 advanced cases treated, there had been just 1 cure and 68 more or less improved. In 188 cases of lupus treated, 7 had considerably improved, 31 had improved, and 30 had died. Overall, just 28 cases could be declared as cures, with nearly 2,000 uncertain or unimproved cases. These were not the results of a successful trial by any means.

That January, even as the experiments continued around the world, the Berlin Medical Society decided that, given the gravity of the disease and the controversy over Koch's cure, some sort of public assessment was in order. The society began a three-month-long debate on tuberculin, with all the Berlin clinicians who were testing it in attendance. Koch himself never appeared; he was, he said, too busy in his laboratory conducting research.

On January 7, 1891, Virchow addressed the society, offering a pathological assessment of Koch's lymph. Inspecting tubercular tissue after a dosage of tuberculin, Virchow detected the dying flesh, or necrosis, that was by now the familiar result of the treatment. But he also clearly detected fresh tubercles, newly sprouted on the edge of the dead tissue. The tuberculin, Virchow suggested, might have some effect on diseased tissue, but it seemed to do nothing whatsoever to abate the actual progress of the disease. Indeed, Virchow argued that the treatment was not only ineffective but also dangerous, and that it likely provoked the spread of the disease.

Virchow's negative assessment proved a turning point. In barely two months, the remedy had gone from a great triumph to occasionally ineffectual to possibly detrimental. Students of Virchow's began referring to the "tuberculin swindle," and Koch was feeling the pressure. On January 15 he at last published a description of tuberculin in general terms: It was, he explained, an extract of dead tuberculosis bacteria mixed in water with an equal part of glycerin. As Koch himself demurred, "My new remedy against tuberculosis is therefore nothing more nor less than a glycerine extract of a pure culture of tubercle bacilli." It seems likely that Koch himself didn't understand how his substance produced a reaction. Still, that reaction was *something*, Koch continued to believe.

By this time, the German government had put the funding for his new institute on hold. The Medical Society's debates continued, casting more doubts on tuberculin and on Koch's entire approach: his premature announcement of a remedy, his poorly designed and supervised experiments, his maneuvering for financial gain, his secrecy. In just two months, the career he'd spent the past fifteen years carefully building seemed to be suspect, his character and his science under assault.

By January 25 the controversy had become overwhelming for Koch. With scarcely any notice, he packed up and left for Egypt on a holiday. The tuberculin experiments were left under the supervision of Eduard Pfuhl, his assistant and son-in-law. He refused to return, he wrote Pfuhl, until funding for a new institute was officially approved. In the meantime, he played the tourist, visiting the ruins of Luxor, exploring the delta north of Cairo, and even getting a suntan. He wrote forlorn letters to Hedwig, his now-eighteen-year-old mistress, calling her by her nickname, Hedchen. "You must know that my discovery has brought out the vultures," he said. "Above all I believe that my work will be successful, but it's going to take a bit of time to prove it. . . . Tell me what you are doing and if you are thinking of me. . . . Dearest Hedchen, if you love me, then I can put up with anything, even failure. Don't leave me now, your love is my comfort and the beacon that guides my path."

He was supposed to be gone for a few weeks. But he wouldn't return to Berlin for three full months.

WE KNOW TODAY THAT KOCH WAS BLINDED BY HIS OWN AMBITION. He so wanted tuberculin to be the cure he sought that he failed to follow his own scientific protocols. In this, he had tripped over one of Sherlock Holmes's maxims: "It is a capital mistake to theorise before one has data. Insensibly one begins to twist facts to suit theories, instead of theories to suit facts."

So why did he overreach? The answer is surely a combination of factors that drove him to put too much faith in too little evidence. There was the pressure from his government, pushing him in August 1890 to make a bold announcement, and then, once he had delivered on its request, pushing him again to turn his preliminary observations into fact. There was Koch's great hunger for his own institute, one designed around his expertise in bacteriology. To that end, tuberculin became his greatest bargaining chip, one that he surely overplayed when he asked to retain monopoly control of the cure and the proceeds from it.

There was also the great competition with Pasteur and legion other scientists. Fifteen years before, the entire field of bacteriology seemed Koch's exclusive domain. But in the years since, it had become the most vibrant area in science, with many ambitious upstarts—most of whom had trained either in his lab or with Pasteur. For all Koch's success in discovery, Pasteur had always bested him when it came to developing therapies, and tuberculin seemed to Koch his best opportunity not only to match his Parisian nemesis, but to outdo him altogether.

And finally, there was young Hedwig. While she worshipped him, she hadn't been around when he was doing his best work. Had tuberculin worked, she would have stood beside him as his reputation, and wealth, soared.

As 1891 wore on, more physicians looked at the numbers and regretted ever having put stock in Koch's remedy. In March, assessing his own experiments with the vaccine, the director of the New York Bacteriological Institute lamented that "we are ... assisting at the spectacle of one of the greatest medical and scientific delusions that has ever existed." At a meeting for internal medicine in Wiesbaden that April, many physicians described their disappointment with Koch's tuberculin in language that sounded like it came from the confession booth. At first, as one doctor described, "the present speaker allowed Koch's discovery to affect him with the full enthusiasm that he was bound to feel. . . . But with the passing of time his self-awareness as a physician increasingly came into conflict with that enthusiasm . . . so that today he no longer dares to use the remedy."

In May, Nicholas Senn, a prominent surgeon in Milwaukee, Wisconsin (and later a president of the American Medical Association), wrote a scathing essay entitled "Away with Koch's Lymph!"

When, six months ago, the telegraph operator at Berlin touched the key of his instrument and flashed to all parts of the civilized world the joyful tidings that a cure for tuberculosis had at last been discovered, the people and the profession felt that the millennium in medicine had come. . . . No other event in the world's history ever attracted so much attention, and no discovery in medicine or surgery ever found such ready introduction and universal acceptation. . . .

Enough time has now elapsed to judge of the merits of the treatment of tuberculosis by Koch's lymph, or, as it is now called, tuberculin. . . . Koch's lymph has been a deceptive bubble which for a short time commanded the attention and admiration of the whole world, but which has been ruthlessly pricked by the critical scalpel.

Dr. Senn's was among the more thorough debunkings of Koch's remedy, and his repugnance was widely shared. Physicians felt they had been duped into dispensing a secret medicine, despite their training that such was anathema to real science. A Berlin physician who had conducted many early tuberculin trials acknowledged that the dubious experiments with the remedy "did not meet the standards of modern science, and its introduction into the sick human body was irresponsible." A German magazine went so far as to suggest that for Koch's next experiment, he should pursue a cure for the "fraud bacillus."

Whispers began circulating: Worse than merely being wrong, Koch had tried to profit from the poor souls with TB. Perhaps, it was rumored, he felt compelled to make money to indulge his young and beautiful girlfriend.

For Koch, the criticism must have been infuriating, particularly considering the praise Pasteur had received after trotting out his vaccines, one after another. Koch, after all, was characteristically the more prudent scientist; he was the more diligent researcher.

That's where Koch caught himself in his own trap—because he himself had used the word *Heilmittel*, "remedy." He had chosen that term, with all its associations, its mystique of health, and its history of false promises. He had offered the ultimate covenant of medicine: that it could undo what nature had done. He had played on his reputation, and the world had taken him at his word. As Harold Ernst, an American physician who visited Berlin, told the Harvard Medical School in January of 1891, before the backlash had turned to outright disgrace, "He is the one man in scientific medicine who thus far has never made a mistake. . . . He is practically the one man by whom the possibility of research in bacteriology has been laid open to us by the development of [his] methods."

Koch had violated the principles that he himself had laid down, his own postulates. Koch had gotten ahead of his evidence. He had made a leap and been caught without a place to land.

AMONG THE MANY IRONIES OF KOCH'S REMEDY WAS THAT IT IN-spired a new wave of false cures. Almost immediately after the No-vember announcement, when demand for the remedy was so great around the world, there were those who peddled concoctions they claimed to be Koch's tuberculin. Then there were the sound-alike medicines: tuberculocidin and tuberculinum and tuberculozyne, tu-berclecide and tuberculoids. Taking a page from Koch, these cures claimed to be "scientific," emerging out of "research laboratories," and "German treatments."

The difference between these quack cures and their sheen of science and Koch's true science was getting lost. The sad coda to the tuberculin fiasco is that over his career, Koch had established a citadel of evidence that proved, as no one had before, that germs are the agent of disease. He had turned that far-fetched idea into a new truth, one that normalized the radicals and marginalized the traditionalists. In the germ theory itself, he had introduced a remedy that was al-ready reducing tuberculosis's deadly hold on the world. And in his discovery of the tuberculosis bacterium, he had shifted the disease from something mysterious and impenetrable into something that could be understood and defended against. That idea, more than any single vaccine or specific treatment, was the real remedy, one that would save millions of lives.

To be sure, the idea of hygiene predated Koch by several decades. In the mid-nineteenth century, hygiene captured the passion of social reformers, who recognized that disease went hand in hand with filth. Edwin Chadwick first captured this spirit in his 1842 report on san-itary conditions in Britain, observing that epidemic and endemic disease "is always found in connexion with the physical circum-stances . . . and where the removal of the noxious agencies appears to be complete, such disease almost entirely disappears."

In 1858, Florence Nightingale built upon Chadwick's observations

...tical analysis of mortality in hospitals. "A vast deal of the
...nd some at least of the mortality, in these establishments is
... Deficient ventilation and over-crowding accompanying
...cts, is to be attributed a large proportion of the evil." Her
conclusions compelled new standards for hospital design and construction. In the 1860s, German science joined the cause, with Virchow
in Berlin and Max von Pettenkofer in Munich advocating massive
new public sanitation projects.

But though their purpose was just and their analysis correct, the
scientific thesis of these hygienists was largely wrong. They fixated on
water and "tainted air" as the agents of disease, rejecting outright any
notion of germs. Nightingale offered a typical argument in 1862:
"What does 'contagion' mean? It implies the communication of
disease from person to person by *contact*. It pre-supposes the existence
of certain germs like the sporules of fungi. . . . There is no end to the
absurdities connected with this doctrine."

What Koch provided through his postulates and his discoveries
was proof, real scientific evidence that germs caused disease. So the
rationale for hygiene was established: Disease-causing germs must be
avoided, rooted out, and eliminated at every opportunity. Moreover,
Koch's evidence was convincing enough to change not just science or
policy, but society itself. He wasn't trading in vague fears about bad
air; he was providing specific causal information about microbes—
with *photographs,* no less.

This specificity provided the leverage for the next wave of reformers to establish social solutions to disease on a vast scale. Where
Pasteur focused on treating individuals, Koch's science led to inter-
ventions on a much broader scale, with the potential to affect and
improve the lives of many more people. Koch's science gave the germ
theory *scale;* it gave it a reach far beyond the laboratory or even the
doctor's office. It moved it into the social realm, where true revolutions happen.

It's hard to overstate the impact of this idea; it transformed the social landscape of everyday experience. In the 1880s and '90s, the water pumps seen throughout most European and American cities became suspect, not only because of the source of the water, but because of the metal cup that was typically chained nearby so that anybody could take a drink from it. Once people realized that germs could spread via the cup, these soon were clipped off (to be replaced, a few years later, with the invention of the disposable paper Dixie cup). People became suspicious of public washrooms. Library books became questionable, since borrowed volumes "may bring the dreaded germs of diphtheria or typhoid fever into homes." Germ theory took such a hold that the New York Public Library assured patrons it would disinfect books periodically, so that "not a live germ can be found." Not even money escaped scrutiny, with "clean money" campaigns catching on worldwide in the 1890s. The New York City Board of Health subsequently analyzed paper currency and coins for bacteria, finding little on coins but thousands of spores on dirty bills. Though the Board of Health found no evidence of "the actual transfer of disease through money," it nonetheless recommended that the US Mint remove old currency from circulation more frequently.

Disinfectants—which had been controversial in hospital operating rooms in the 1860s, when Lister first proposed them—began to be used in ordinary households. The first, appropriately, was called Listerine. Invented in 1879 by a St. Louis doctor as a surgery disinfectant, it was later sold as a floor cleaner and treatment for venereal diseases (and later still, for halitosis). Ivory soap, one of Procter and Gamble's first products, went on the market in 1879 and was soon followed by other soaps and disinfectants. In 1882, New York's Casper Cohn started selling Germicide, an apparatus for delivering a proprietary blend of a bacteria-killing formula; his first brochure noted that "although the reception of the germ theory of disease has been gradual, it may now be said to be clearly established in the public mind."

Robert Koch can also be thanked for helping to curb the habit of

spitting. Before his discoveries, spitting was thought to be merely uncouth. But after he established that contagious germs could be passed
via saliva, the habit was seen as downright dangerous. An 1882 essay
in *Modern Medicine and Bacteriological World* made it seem yet more
malevolent:

> The man who hawks on the street and constantly clears his
> throat in company, or expectorates indiscriminately, whether
> walking or sitting is surely an object of dread to all refined
> natures, if not an actual menace to public health in general. I
> have known one pachydermatous individual, who was suf-
> fering with lung trouble, and yet thoughtless enough to foist
> his undesirable presence on a group of men, quickly clear a
> room or office of his erst-while sympathizers by coughing,
> hawking, and spitting in a handy spittoon.

Soon this disdain began to coalesce into a campaign. Citing "the
correctness of Koch's theory" in 1885, Dr. J. M. Emmert, the president
of the Iowa State Board of Health, urged that a broad new antispitting
social policy be enacted. "How necessary it is," he argued, "to prevent
the spitting by tuberculous persons upon the streets, in stores, hotels,
depots, railway cars, in fact anywhere and everywhere."

In cities and nations, there were growing campaigns against
spitting, turning tolerance into revulsion. In France, this was girded
in the tenor of war. "Le crachat, voilà l'ennemi!" ("Spitting, that is the
enemy!") one French periodical told its readers. "Each *crachat* is, alas!
a veritable army of billions of vigorous microbes, that [one] sends to
attack the health of [one's] wife, children, friends, and neighbors."

In American cities, antispitting associations began to form,
calling on politicians to outlaw public expectoration and posting signs
chastising spitters—"Spitting is DANGEROUS and ILLEGAL!"—
in rail stations and other public spaces. In 1896, New York City passed
an antispitting statute (the predecessor to today's bans on cigarettes

and Big Gulps), and the next year, ordinances were passed in Rochester, New York, and Columbus, Ohio. Soon most major cities in the United States had outlawed public expectoration.

IN 1892 THE FIRST ORGANIZATION DEDICATED TO THE ERADICATION of tuberculosis was formed in Pennsylvania; within twenty years, nearly every major city and every European nation had a similar group, dedicated to destroying the disease through not the application of a specific drug or treatment, but the dissemination of information. In fact, the campaign against TB would be the first mass health education campaign directed at one disease. Not just a campaign of doctors and scientists, it would soon recruit the whole of society, from US presidents to housewives. Koch's germ theory was changing behavior at every level of society. He'd convinced science and society that germs could be lethal and that if we avoided the bad ones, we could avoid disease.

In August 1892, Koch finally had a chance to demonstrate this himself, when the city of Hamburg, in northern Germany, experienced a violent cholera outbreak. In the space of a few weeks, more than seventeen thousand cases and eight thousand deaths were reported, causing a national panic. Koch arrived and soon began looking in the water for the telltale bacterium, the same one he'd identified years before in India. He soon found it festering in the city's aboveground water supply. The next question was how to keep the disease from returning. Koch showed that a belowground supply would provide a natural sand filter that screened out the microbe. Based on this work, the German government required all municipalities to examine the sources of their water supply and apply filters where necessary.

To see disease in order to stop it: This principle had perhaps its greatest champion in Hermann Biggs. While a student at New York City's Bellevue Medical College, Biggs was taught by William Henry

Welch, who had the good fortune of working in Koch's Berlin laboratory in 1885. (Welch would go on to be one of the most famous physicians in the United States.) In 1882, when Koch discovered the *Mycobacterium tuberculosis*, Welch impressed upon his students, including Biggs, the significance of the discovery. A decade later, in 1892, Biggs opened a new bacteriological laboratory for the New York City Department of Health, modeled on Koch's own laboratory principles. Just weeks after opening the lab, Biggs began racking up triumphs, including detecting cholera on a newly arrived ship of immigrants (their quarantine prevented an outbreak spreading in the city) and, in 1893, locking down a Russian ship contaminated with typhus.

In 1894, Biggs wrote a polemic, "To Rob Consumption of Its Terrors." Even with the disaster of tuberculin fresh in medical minds, Biggs reminded readers of the importance of Koch's original discovery. "The knowledge we now have of the causation of tuberculosis makes possible the formulation of perfectly efficient means for its prevention." Biggs recommended a municipally driven system of education, segregation, and disinfection, with a great increase in the number of sanitariums, for both isolation and recovery. With these measures, Biggs believed, "we have it in our power to completely wipe out pulmonary tuberculosis in a single generation."

By 1897, New York City had passed an ordinance requiring the mandatory reporting of tuberculosis cases in the city. Soon Biggs had a map of disease in Manhattan as powerful as John Snow's cholera map of London. No longer a disease lurking in the shadows, TB, as Biggs showed, could be counted, tracked, evaluated, and combated.

Though governments rarely went as far as Biggs would have them, in record books from Paris to New York to London, a pronounced drop-off in tuberculosis cases can be traced to the 1880s, when Koch's discovery began to spread. In New York, fatalities from pulmonary tuberculosis had hovered around four hundred per hundred thousand annually for most of the nineteenth century. But beginning in 1880, that rate began to drop precipitously, to three hundred per hundred thousand in 1890 and one hundred per hundred thousand by 1920. By 1950, when the first antibiotics effective against the disease were developed, the rate was already down to a mere twenty-seven per hundred thousand. Other cities that embraced hygiene experienced a similar drop-off; deaths in Paris, for instance, fell from five hundred per hundred thousand in 1870 to three hundred per hundred thousand in 1910.

Tuberculin may not have led to the glory Koch yearned for, but thanks to people such as Hermann Biggs, who took Koch's ideas and built on them, Koch's science became a kind of remedy nonetheless.

IN MAY OF 1891 THE GERMAN GOVERNMENT AT LAST APPROVED funding for Koch's Institute for Infectious Diseases. As the institute's director, Koch was granted the salary of twenty thousand marks—not the fortune he may have expected from tuberculin, but a robust salary nonetheless.

This time, though, there would be no profit from discoveries and no covert experimentation. "There must be no more secrecy," insisted a member of the German parliament during the funding debate. "There must be no more experimenting on human bodies with a secret remedy." The deal required Koch to agree that any inventions or discoveries "would be placed unconditionally and without any compensation whatsoever at the government's disposal." In addition, it required him to come clean on tuberculin and deliver a full analysis of its chemical composition before he could take his new post. (He would publish a full accounting of tuberculin that fall.)

With that, the next chapter of Koch's life began. In 1892 he was officially divorced. He married Hedwig, nearly thirty years his junior, in September 1893—three years after he'd first met her.

At the new institute, Koch's subordinates began to take center stage. In 1893, Paul Ehrlich and Emil von Behring began to investigate an antitoxin for diphtheria, a dangerous bacterial infection that caused severe respiratory distress. It typically occurred in epidemics, often killing hundreds of children in an outbreak. Von Behring would independently develop and perfect the serum in 1894 (much to Ehrlich's dismay). Meanwhile, Ehrlich would continue to investigate how the body produces antibodies and how it develops immunity to disease, the basis for our conception of the immune system.

It was this notion of an immune system that Koch lacked in his analysis of tuberculin. Today we understand that the substance was, in fact, causing an immune response in the body. Koch mistook a *reaction* for a *remedy,* and that mistake was everything.

As the decade progressed, Koch became more and more detached from the work at his institute, until his role was largely ceremonial. In 1895, word came from Paris that Louis Pasteur, his great rival for more than fifteen years, had died. In 1896, Koch and his young wife set off for South Africa, this time to begin a years-long investigation of tropical diseases: mainly malaria and sleeping sickness. At the time, critics gossiped that he was leaving Germany to escape the dual disgrace of tuberculin and divorce. In truth, however, he was leaving at the behest of the German government, which increasingly saw infectious disease as an enemy to the growing empire and Koch as its field general. Whatever the impetus, Koch seemed to be more than willing to leave his laboratory behind. Now in his midfifties, he was following the dream he'd had as a teenager back in Clausthal. He was following the path of von Humboldt, exploring the world.

CHAPTER 9

1892 · The Rise of A. C. Doyle

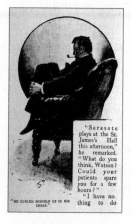

"Sarasate plays at the St. James's Hall this afternoon," he remarked. "What do you think, Watson? Could your patients spare you for a few hours?"
"I have nothing to do

"HE CURLED HIMSELF UP IN HIS CHAIR."

Holmes at work, an illustration by Sidney Paget from
"The Red-Headed League," published in The Strand, *August 1891*

Arthur Conan Doyle arrived back in Southsea on November 22, 1890, both exhausted and elated. He had done it.

Entirely on impulse, he had set off to an unfamiliar city (without a single contact or connection), successfully witnessed (albeit by proxy) one of the most significant scientific demonstrations of the past fifty years, and then had the wherewithal to beat every journalist and every physician in Europe to evaluate the evidence. Koch's remedy may have gestured at a revolution, Conan Doyle recognized, but it could not deliver one—and he was likely the first person in the world to say as much.

"I came back a changed man," he later recalled in his memoirs. "I had spread my wings and had felt something of the powers within me." Once back in Southsea, he wasted no time in cutting the cord. "I am leaving Southsea shortly," he told the *Portsmouth Evening Mail* on November 24, just two days after his return from Berlin. "I am going to Vienna in January. I shall remain for three months to study the eye after which I intend to start in London as a specialist." His plan followed Dr. Morris's prescription precisely. And indeed, by December 18, Conan Doyle had sold his practice and left Southsea forever.

By January, when skepticism about Koch's remedy was rising in Berlin, Conan Doyle was a world away, in Vienna, with Touie. (They had left two-year-old daughter Mary with Touie's mother on the Isle of Wight.) They arrived during a snowstorm, on a bitterly cold night, "a gloomy, ominous reception," Conan Doyle noted. And it didn't get much better from there.

The couple quickly found room in a pleasant pension on Universitätesstrasse, one of Vienna's main streets, for four pounds a week. During the days, Conan Doyle attended lectures at the university, but the language was a problem. Though he spoke German well thanks to his year in high school in Austria, he found the technical terminology of the classroom and laboratory frustrating, and he struggled to keep up. Not that he was terribly dedicated to his studies, anyway. In the afternoons, rather than study his ophthalmology texts, he would sit down at his desk and write stories. His output was prodigious: He finished a novel, *The Doings of Raffles Haw,* a tale about a man who discovers how to manufacture gold (he dedicated it to Dr. Morris); wrote a first draft of *The Refugees,* a novel set in the time of Louis XIV, which he sold for serialization in the American magazine *Harper's;* and turned out several shorter stories, including one titled "The Voice of Science." He sold that to a new monthly magazine in London called *The Strand.*

The couple did their best to enjoy Vienna. They did some sightseeing, went ice-skating, and splurged on the Anglo-American Ball. But Conan Doyle soon grew impatient. Dr. Morris had suggested he spend six months in Vienna, but barely eight weeks passed before he and Touie packed up and left. They stopped for a week in Paris, where Conan Doyle spent some time with the French opthalmologist Edmond Landolt—he would later exaggerate these visits into full-fledged studies in Paris—and then were back in England by late March.

In London, the Conan Doyles let a flat on Montague Place, in the shadow of the great British Museum. For a consulting room, Conan Doyle went to Regent's Park, a neighborhood popular with prominent physicians, and rented an office at 2 Devonshire Place (just a few blocks from Baker Street, as it happens). Expectations were great—"our boats were burned behind us," Conan Doyle wrote in a letter—but patients failed to materialize. Every morning, he would arrive at his office and sit there expectantly. At three or four in the afternoon he would put on his coat and walk back to Montague Place. Day after day the bell never rang, which gave him more time to write at a furious pace. And as Conan Doyle considered his commercial opportunities and the literary landscape, he hatched an idea for a new sort of story. Monthly magazines remained the most promising and lucrative forum for his work, but he had tired of writing novels for serialization. Strung out so, serialized fiction seemed padded, even aimless, and too dependent on dedicated readers who would devotedly buy every issue. Perhaps, Conan Doyle thought, a new structure could take advantage of the monthly format but not punish any readers for missing an installment: a series of independent stories that featured one recurring character. Each story would be self-contained, with a satisfying resolution, but the main protagonist would appear in each one.

Then he realized he already had the perfect character for such an experiment: Sherlock Holmes. Within a week of setting up in London, the first Holmes short story, "A Scandal in Bohemia," was off to Conan Doyle's agent; from there, it went on to *The Strand Magazine*.

The Strand seemed the ideal venue for the experiment. Published by George Newnes, who promised readers that it would "cost sixpence and be worth a shilling," *The Strand* was aimed at a more upmarket crowd than Newnes's thriving middle-of-the-road weekly, *Tit-Bits*. It took the bold step of including an illustration on every page, a pioneering use of artwork. Herbert Greenhough Smith, *The Strand*'s editor, accepted the story and asked Conan Doyle for more. "There was no mistaking the ingenuity of the plot, the limpid clearness of the style, the perfect art of telling a story," Greenhough Smith said later, noting that it "brought a gleam of happiness into the despairing life of this weary editor."

Over time, Conan Doyle honed a precise method for crafting a Holmes story. He would sit down at his desk, writing paper stacked neatly to one side, the oil lamp lit on the other, and notebooks at hand with ideas or sketches. He would first structure the story, starting with the solution to a crime. Working backward, he would chart the clues, setting them out in a certain order, the chain of evidence that would slowly accumulate in the telling. He would have to make sure Holmes didn't benefit unfairly from his vantage point; the clues would have to be real. At the same time, he couldn't allow a mystery to be too easy for readers to solve before Holmes brandished his own brilliant solution. There would be real clues, and some facts that seemed like clues but were extraneous to where the story was leading. Only Conan Doyle would know which was which, and Holmes's only advantage was his method.

Each story was a puzzle that Conan Doyle had to assemble carefully, but the method let him work quickly; a tale took him no more than a week. And once he laid it out, Conan Doyle wouldn't consider going back to revise or edit his prose. Any such improvements, he felt, would be "gratuitous and a waste of time." The stories were slotted to begin appearing in *The Strand* that summer, and Conan Doyle enjoyed the sublime feeling of being on top of his game.

And then, one May morning a few days shy of his thirty-third birthday, Conan Doyle was making his early jaunt from Montague Street to Devonshire Place when suddenly he was overcome by a severe chill. It shook him to his bones, and he felt all at once horribly ill. He turned around and retraced his steps, struggling to reach his home on Montague. He went immediately to bed and would not rise again for days. He had come down with a severe case of influenza.

The disease was not to be taken lightly. His sister Annette had died of the flu just sixteen months earlier. As it happened, 1891, when Conan Doyle was struck, turned out to be a particularly deadly year for flu; nearly seventeen thousand Britons would die of the illness, four times as many as in the prior year.

Conan Doyle was in great danger for a week, and it would be several weeks before he was up on his feet, hobbling about with a walking stick. Yet the convalescence provided him with an opportunity to take stock. He considered his half measure of moving to London to pursue ophthalmology and writing on the side. Perhaps it was all wrong, a too-timid assessment of his potential. His literary career, he realized, was thriving, while his medical career was, for all purposes, nonexistent. Indeed, while literature was providing him with a comfortable income, medicine was only costing him money. His heart, he realized, was no longer in it.

For Conan Doyle, the moment came as an epiphany and a profound feeling of utter liberation. "It was one of the great moments of exultation of my life," he recalled later. It was the second time in a year that infectious disease would provoke a profound shift in Conan Doyle's life. By the end of June, he had given up medicine for good. Once again, he loaded up the family's belongings, for the third time in six months, and headed for South Norwood, a neighborhood south of London. He packed away his microscope, his stethoscope, and his other instruments, rarely to use them again.

Conan Doyle had gotten a great deal out of medicine: an education, a sense of stature and accomplishment, and most of all a worldview. His was by now a thoroughly scientific mind, whether or not he still chose to participate in that science. Medical science informed how he thought; it influenced how he wrote; and quite clearly it was inseparable from *what* he wrote. "I can testify how great a privilege and how valuable a possession it is to be a medical man, and to have had a medical training, even though one does not use it," he remarked later. He didn't need to practice medicine anymore. He didn't need to pretend that he wanted a successful medical career. He could finally say that he had, at last, surpassed the dream he'd described to his mother fifteen years prior: a thriving practice, a surgical appointment, and some stories on the side. The stories, he could now admit, were everything.

In the first days of July, three hundred thousand copies of *The Strand* began to appear in shops around Britain. They were soon all sold out, the public captivated by the tale of that consulting detective. *The Book Buyer* magazine proclaimed that "Whoever sets sail on a voyage of discovery with Dr. Conan Doyle may fairly expect that romance will preside at the helm." Such sentiments pleased Conan Doyle—especially since they recognized him as a writer of literature, first and foremost. He was now a man with a reputation, a following, and a steady income.

Why did these stories captivate the public's imagination when the two previous novels had not? What had changed in the five years since 1886, when *A Study in Scarlet* had made scarcely a ripple in the public's mind? For one thing, *The Strand* editors recognized the power of images, and they had lavishly illustrated the stories with drawings by Sidney Paget. Paget wasn't the first choice; the commission was intended for his brother Walter, who had previously illustrated Robert Louis Stevenson's *Treasure Island* and *Robinson Crusoe*. But the end result was inspired. Paget adroitly captured Conan Doyle's description of Holmes's profile: the beaked nose, sharp chin, and lean build. But Paget's Holmes is more elegant and less odd than Conan Doyle describes. He appears handsome, well-dressed, and neat—a worthy hero, in other words, not the drug-addled malcontent of *The Sign of Four*. It was Paget, not Conan Doyle, who outfitted Holmes in his trademark cape and deerstalker hat. The drawings soon became an essential part of *The Strand*'s dramatic layout, and the magazine often devoted an entire page to at least one illustration.

The shorter form, too, made for a brisker pace and a faster plot. "A Scandal in Bohemia," at just over eight thousand words, streaks from Prague to Warsaw and back to Baker Street. The mysteries, too, were more than routine potboiler detective tales. The central case in "A Scandal in Bohemia" does not concern a murder, but rather a lost photograph—a much subtler sort of intrigue. The second story, "The Red-Headed League," involves an ingenious plot about a criminal gang that wants to tunnel into a bank through a shop; to get the shop owner and his "blazing red head" out of the premises, they place a newspaper advertisement offering four pounds a week to all members of the Red-Headed League. Holmes sorts out the case with a flourish.

But the appeal probably lay most of all in Holmes himself, and his odd combination of zeal and insouciance. By now Conan Doyle had all but perfected the routine: The oddly cold and calculating detective is called, takes the laboratory into the streets, and turns the power of science toward the everyday mysteries of murder and intrigue. Holmes is precise, methodical, and keenly perceptive. He ably appropriates the techniques of the bacteriologist to discern what seems otherwise invisible. As he says in "A Case of Identity," "it has long been an axiom of mine that the little things are infinitely more important." This is Sherlock Holmes's singular quality, and it was particularly well suited to the age.

By 1891, science was no longer seen as some radical challenge to European culture; instead, it seemed in many ways to *define* the culture. This was true in Germany and France and especially in Britain, where science seemed to touch something in the Victorian spirit. As a speech published in the British science journal *Nature* put it in 1890, "Ours would be remembered as pre-eminently the age of science. Our successors might excel us as writers, as politicians, as soldiers; they might surpass even the industrial energies of the present time, but it was not likely—it was scarcely possible—that in the region of science the twentieth century should witness advances greater than, or as great as, those of the nineteenth."

As Europe raced toward the twentieth century, science became an outright fad, the prism through which the rest of the culture viewed itself (not unlike technology today). The popular literature was filled with scientific stories, among them Robert Louis Stevenson's *Strange Case of Dr. Jekyll and Mr. Hyde,* and most of all those of H. G. Wells, who in the course of ten years wrote *The Time Machine, The Island of Doctor Moreau, The Invisible Man,* and *War of the Worlds.* But even Wells himself, in an essay titled "Popularising Science," published in the journal *Nature* in 1894, acknowledged that it was Conan Doyle, through his character Sherlock Holmes, who had best captured this spirit. The Holmes stories, Wells wrote, "show that the public delights in the ingenious unraveling of evidence, and Conan Doyle need never stoop to jesting. First the problem, then the gradual piecing together of the solution. They cannot get enough of such matter."

Part of Holmes's appeal was that his science wasn't mere erudition. Rather, he applied it always with utility and purpose, with tangible rewards and results. When he turned his magnifying glass upon footprints or his microscope on tobacco ash, he typified the pragmatic spirit of the age. At last science was revealing a more immediate world, one that had profound human consequences.

For contemporary observers, Holmes's debt to science was unmistakable. "Holmes is a true product of his time," an 1896 literary review stated. "He is an embodiment of the scientific spirit seeing microscopically and applying itself to construct, from material vestiges and psychologic remainders, an unknown body of proof."

Scientists, too, found Holmes's methods captivating, and the detective a worthy representative of their work. A 1903 textbook titled

The Teaching of Scientific Method recommended that budding researchers "read *The Memoirs of Sherlock Holmes*, by Conan Doyle, and see how, by noticing a number of small signs, he 'puts this and that together' and gathers important information. This, again, is precisely our method—the scientific method."

Even the bacteriologists back in Germany adored Holmes and his creator. Paul Ehrlich reportedly filled the margins of Holmes stories with comments and formulas. When Conan Doyle heard that Ehrlich was a fan, he sent him a note of appreciation and a signed photograph, which Ehrlich proudly hung on the wall in his study.

Conan Doyle may have found Koch's remedy wanting, but he had learned something in Berlin, watching the consumptive masses stream into the city: how much people now expected of science, how much the public was open to its power to improve their lives. Conan Doyle's great insight was to see that openness as an opportunity to turn science into entertainment.

By September 1891, when Conan Doyle delivered the sixth Holmes story to *The Strand*, it was clear that he had a phenomenon on his hands. On the day a new story was due, readers would queue up in front of shops, waiting for the magazine issue to be delivered. Many readers assumed Sherlock Holmes was real and went on pilgrimages to Baker Street, only to find there was no such address as 221b. Conan Doyle was buried in fan mail, with many correspondents asking for an autograph from Sherlock Holmes. Even his mother asked him to sign a note for a friend using the name "Sherlock Holmes," a request Conan Doyle took as the worst possible insult. Not even his mother, of all people, could distinguish between the fictional character and his flesh-and-blood creator. Others proposed plots for the next mystery, and some wrote to Holmes asking the fictional detective to take up their own case of missing relatives or pets. *Strand* editor George Newnes estimated that having Conan Doyle's name on the cover of his magazine ensured he would sell a hundred thousand more copies. Greenhough Smith quickly commissioned six more stories from the writer.

Conan Doyle soon finished up the series and spent the next year away from his detective. Instead, he embraced his status as one of England's most popular authors. Friendships with other authors— among them James Barrie, author of *Peter Pan*, and Bram Stoker, author of *Dracula*—followed. His family life was comfortable, even leisurely.

The only wrinkle came with Touie, whose gentle disposition seemed perhaps somewhat more vulnerable. She was afflicted, as they said then, with a weak constitution. Always a vigorous sportsman himself, Conan Doyle would coax her to join him on bicycle rides, and they'd venture into the countryside on the new tandem cycle he'd splurged on. But Touie was quick to tire. On one such jaunt into the country, she made it only halfway, returning home by train. She slept often, and while she insisted to her husband that she was happy, she seemed deeply sad.

In October 1892, the first twelve Holmes stories were collected in book form as *The Adventures of Sherlock Holmes*. It was an immediate bestseller, with nearly 250,000 copies sold over the next three years. Considering how long Conan Doyle had worked for success and acclaim—he had now been writing professionally for nearly fifteen years—it's rather remarkable how quickly he came to quibble with it. He wanted to be recognized as a serious literary author, not a peddler of mere detective stories. Too many of the letters he received in South Norwood were to Holmes, he complained, not to him, a mistake Conan Doyle took as an insult instead of a testament to the power of his imagination. As early as November 1891, he complained to his mother that the detective was a distraction, referring to Holmes almost as a real person. "I think of slaying Holmes . . . and winding him up for good and all. He takes my mind from better things."

She was aghast. "You can't! You won't! You mustn't!" She admired the stories but was also offended that he would deprive his family of such an opportunity.

He assured her he would keep at it. "He still lives," he wrote her the next January, "thanks to your entreaties."

In early 1892, Greenhough Smith asked—begged, really—for a second series of Holmes stories. By this point, Conan Doyle had had a few months off from the demands of crafting a Holmes story, but the thought of it, he said, made him nearly physically sick. He wanted to move on to the real literature he was capable of, the stuff he'd written in *The White Company* and *Micah Clarke*. This was the work Conan Doyle was proud of; instead, he was being pushed backward toward more detective yarns.

He considered turning Greenhough Smith down outright, but pragmatism got the better of him. He suggested what seemed like an outrageous proposal: twelve stories for a thousand pounds. It was an unheard-of sum, and he expected the request would be quickly rejected, allowing him to move on. No such luck: Greenhough Smith quickly agreed. Conan Doyle was back on the hook for more Holmes.

The second series began with "The Adventure of Silver Blaze," which appeared in *The Strand* in December 1892, followed by other stories monthly. Conan Doyle was nearly done writing them when, in July 1893, he and Touie left for a holiday in Switzerland. The official purpose was a lecture in Lucerne, but Conan Doyle hoped, too, that they could spend some time in the mountains, which might restore Touie's health. She had seemed in particularly poor spirits, with little energy or enthusiasm ever since their son, Kinglsey, was born the previous November. The mountain air, Conan Doyle hoped, would benefit her.

One morning, Conan Doyle left Touie at their hotel and went on a ramble with some friends. The destination was Meiringen, in the Bernese Alps. They climbed a ridge and came upon Reichenbach Falls, a cascading series of waterfalls with a total drop of 250 meters, or more than 800 feet. "The torrent, swollen by the melting snow, plunges into a tremendous abyss," Conan Doyle later described, "from which the spray rolls up like the smoke from a burning house." He gazed down at the falls, taking in the violence below, and he knew, almost instantly that this would be a "worthy tomb" for Holmes, "even if I buried my bank account along with him."

Back in South Norwood, he began writing the tale, the last installment in *The Strand*'s second series. "I am in the middle of the last Holmes story," he wrote his mother, "after which the gentleman vanishes, never to return. I am weary of his name." Finally, one evening, he sat down at his desk, opened his diary, and wrote just two words: "Killed Holmes."

In the fall of 1893, Touie's health took a bad turn. She began to cough constantly and sometimes violently, forcing up mucus tinged with blood. With every breath, a coarse crackle resounded deep in her chest, like a wet log cast onto a hot fire. Her side began to hurt, an ache that no amount of bed rest seemed to lessen. These were unmistakable symptoms, the all-too-routine indications of an all-too-common disease. This was consumption, plain as day.

Perhaps Conan Doyle had seen the signs for years and denied them; perhaps he believed that Touie simply had a weak constitution. Regardless, whatever he had missed before was now manifest. One day, when she couldn't leave bed for coughing so hard, Conan Doyle sent for a doctor. He arrived at the house in South Norwood, spoke with Conan Doyle, and then went upstairs to see Touie. Conan Doyle stayed downstairs, and after what seemed like an eternity, the doctor came back down looking stern. His verdict: galloping consumption.

"To my surprise and alarm he told me when he descended from the bedroom that the lungs were very gravely affected, that there was every sign of rapid consumption and that he thought the case a most serious one with little hope, considering her record and family history, of a permanent cure." Not yet prepared to face a disease with no real remedy, a few days later Conan Doyle sent for a second doctor, "one of the first men in London." The second opinion was the same as the first. "He seemed to think that the mischief must have been going on for years unobserved," Conan Doyle wrote his mother, telling her the sad news. "The cough is occasionally troublesome & the phlegm very thick—no hemmhorrhage yet, but I fear it."

Of all diseases, it had to be tuberculosis—this most tenacious of infections, one that Conan Doyle was well familiar with. This same affliction had drawn him to Berlin, a trip that inspired him to break free of medicine. And now tuberculosis was back in his life.

However close Conan Doyle had been to tuberculosis scientifically, he couldn't quite fathom it coming so close to him personally. Despite the years he'd admired Koch's work, despite his investigations in Berlin just two years prior, he had missed the clues right in front of him. But Conan Doyle was never a man for second thoughts. Within the week, he'd begun making arrangements to give up the house in South Norwood, sell the furniture, and leave for Davos, Switzerland, home of the most famous tuberculosis hospitals in Europe. By early November, Touie had arrived at the Kurhaus Hotel, a favorite retreat for well-off English consumptives. For his part, Conan Doyle had a series of lectures around Europe; he would arrive in Davos in early December.

Conan Doyle didn't choose the Brompton Hospital in London, still the most celebrated consumptive hospital in England. And he didn't place his hopes on chemical cures or treatments. If there was any hope of improvement, it was in the dry mountain climate of the Alps. And not once did Conan Doyle even seem to consider that supposed cure, tuberculin. In all his letters and recollections, Koch's remedy never appears to have come up.

THE STORY WAS ENTITLED "THE ADVENTURE OF THE FINAL Problem" (later shortened to "The Final Problem"). In it, Holmes and

Watson travel to Switzerland, hoping to snare Holmes's nemesis, Professor Moriarty. A man of fierce intellect put to nefarious purposes, Moriarty is "the organizer of half that is evil and of nearly all that is undetected in this great city," as Holmes describes him to Watson. Still, Holmes can't help but admire Moriarty: "He is a genius, a philosopher, an abstract thinker. He has a brain of the first order." The story, in fact, isn't a mystery at all, insofar as there is any detective work or deduction. Rather, Conan Doyle presents it as a kind of coda, Watson's personal explanation of the great detective's last days. He includes a curious detail to the story: While climbing up to the Reichenbach Falls with Holmes, Watson is met by a man from their hotel; an Englishwoman there is deathly ill with consumption. She had just left Davos, he is told, when "a sudden hemorrhage had overtaken her," and she demanded an English doctor.

There is no sick woman, however. The message is just a ruse by Moriarty to get the great detective alone. With Watson out of the way, Moriarty races up the cliff to confront Sherlock Holmes, they tussle, and then both tumble over the side, into the falls, to their mutual and certain death.

When the story appeared in mid-December, in *The Strand*'s Christmas double issue, it caused an immediate reaction bordering on scandal. In London, men reportedly wore black armbands. Women wrote outraged letters. "You brute!" one chastised Conan Doyle. *The Literary News* took the tidings with umbrage: Conan Doyle may have invented the character, they felt, but Holmes was not entirely his. "What excuse Dr. Doyle can present for such summary exhaustion of this rich mine of adventure is hard to conceive. Dr. Doyle may have become tired of Holmes, but his readers have not."

The Strand received bushels of angry correspondence and lost twenty thousand readers. The magazine tried to stand with its audience. "Like hundreds of correspondents, we feel as if we have lost an old friend whom we could ill spare." The editors promised that

more stories would appear shortly, after "only a temporary interval."
But it was wishful thinking. For years afterward, the story recounting
Holmes's death would be known in *The Strand* offices as "the Dreadful
Event."

But Conan Doyle was no longer in London to witness the outrage;
by this time he had arrived in Davos to care for his sick wife. After a
few weeks in Switzerland, Touie seemed somewhat improved. She
had gained back some weight and some cheer. While she rested in the
hotel, Conan Doyle tried his hand at winter sports. When descriptions of the reaction back in England reached him, he was embarrassed, even flummoxed. It was more than he'd expected, to be honest,
and he wondered a little what it was about Holmes that proved so
damned appealing. Frankly, he had felt no alternative. In an 1894 interview with *The Bookman*, an American journal, he defended himself.
"I have come to take you in custody for the killing of Sherlock
Holmes," his interviewer said when they sat down.

"Ah, but I did it in self-defense," he replied. "And if you knew
the provocation you would agree with me that it was justifiable homicide. When I invented this character I had no idea
he would give me so much trouble. But when 'Holmes' Adventures' began to appear in the Strand Magazine, its circulation went up by leaps and bounds until it reached the
phenomenal figure of four hundred thousand. No sooner had
one story appeared than I was set upon for another, and such
considerable sums of money were offered by the publishers, in-
dicating a popular demand so imperative and so flattering,
that I was tempted repeatedly from other work which I greatly
desired to finish. I went on from one case to another until, as
you know, there are now two volumes of the Memoirs and
Adventures of Sherlock Holmes. At last I killed him, and . . .
if I had not done so I almost think he would have killed me."

That was that. He was done with Holmes. His attentions were back on tuberculosis, where they had been two years earlier in Berlin. Back then, the horrific power and tenacity of the microbe served as an intellectual puzzle, requiring him to apply both his scientific training and his gift for words to explain to the world why this tiny germ was impervious to the great Robert Koch's cure. But now, Conan Doyle felt the bacterium's nastiness firsthand. He could see how it devoured hope and left only helplessness. He pined for some sort of cure, even as he knew how impossible one would be. His mind went back to the riddles of bacteriology and how geniuses such as Koch had failed to sleuth their way to a remedy.

"What an infernal microbe it is!" he wrote to a friend back in England. "Surely science will find some way of destroying it. How absurd that we who can kill the tiger should be defied by this venomous little atom. . . . They gnaw at you as cheesemites do into cheese. . . . Could we not impregnate every tissue of the body so that they could not live?"

CHAPTER 10

1900 · The New Century

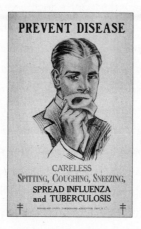

A poster campaign to stop tuberculosis, circa 1925

Koch's arrival in South Africa in December 1896 was well-timed. A plague of rinderpest was taking a deadly toll on the nation's cattle, and Koch was greeted like a hero come to save the day. He was flattered and impressed by the faith the local medical community placed in science. "In Europe," he remarked to the audience, "it was never very easy to persuade people to . . . utilize modern science." He was ever the faithful rationalist.

Koch spent a year and a half in South Africa, working on a rudimentary rinderpest vaccine. Then he and Hedwig were off to India to investigate an outbreak of bubonic plague, and then to German East Africa (now Tanzania, Burundi, and Rwanda) to tackle plague and malaria. Malaria took him next to the Dutch East Indies (today's Indonesia), then under German control. Koch spent nearly a year there, formulating a new method for the control of malaria based on the therapeutic and prophylactic use of quinine. His technique captured no headlines, but it would remain the world standard for more than forty years.

He spent nearly four years on these journeys, with only a brief return to Berlin. Despite the months-long ocean voyages and days of waiting in port for the next passage, he took to the sojourns as a relief. He was, in part, running away from the mess he had created in Berlin. But he also saw Africa as an opportunity, a place where he could once again simply pursue science. "At home," he wrote an old colleague, "there are so many demands on my time, and controversies are so fierce, that it is virtually impossible to get any work done. Out here in Africa, one can find bits of scientific gold lying on the streets."

In 1900, Koch finally returned to Berlin to accept the appointment as director of a new Institute for Infectious Diseases. (The previous institute, established after the frenzy over tuberculin, had become too small for the demands of modern microbiology.) This would be his final official affiliation in Berlin. The designation was largely honorary; he appeared to have no official administrative or scientific duties. But at this new institute, as before, he would have a personal lab to carry out his own work. There, perhaps, he could rebuild his reputation and return to the serious study of microorganisms and disease.

Then tuberculosis, Koch's great nemesis and accomplice at once, again demanded his attention. In July 1901 he was invited to London to attend the British Congress of Tuberculosis, conceived as an international assessment of the battle against TB as the new century dawned. Though there had been much research since Koch's great discovery of the bacilli twenty years earlier, true progress toward cures or treatments had been disappointing. But there was hope in hygiene, especially in new ideas about preventive measures between animals and humans, where it was suspected many cases of the disease began.

As far as the congress organizers were concerned, Koch's presence was largely ceremonial, a nod to his original discovery of the bacilli. But Koch had other ideas. On the first day, he received a medal for his contributions to science and then was invited to the podium to deliver some remarks. His topic was the relationship between human and bovine tuberculosis. Since his 1882 discovery, it was widely known that cows, as well as humans, suffered from something like tuberculosis. Building on the germ theory, most scientists believed that cows could be a vector for the human disease, the bacteria passing through the milk of an infected animal. This theory seemed in keeping with Koch's work, since it traced a specific trajectory from animals to humans. It was bolstered by the discovery of a mycobacterium in cows in 1898.

As Koch began his remarks, though, the audience seemed baffled by his flow of thought. Instead of endorsing a link between the human and bovine diseases, Koch's language went the other way, until it dawned on the crowd that Koch, remarkably, was outright denying any connection between the two diseases. He had inspected the bovine bacterium, he said, and found it altogether unlike the human bacterium he had isolated twenty years earlier. Therefore, he said, there could be no connection. As for any preventive measures aimed at intercepting the spread of tuberculosis from cows to people, he considered them altogether useless. "I should estimate the extent of infection by the milk and flesh of tubercular cattle and the butter made of their milk as hardly greater than that of hereditary trans-mission," he said, knowing full well that the disease's bacteriological nature made hereditary transmission impossible. "I therefore do not deem it advisable to take any measures against it."

His remarks couldn't have been more disruptive than if he'd re-nounced the germ theory altogether. Here was Koch, the great vi-sionary, denying a link that dozens of other scientists—*building on Koch's own work*—had validated. The claim drew immediate retorts, with von Behring the most vocal. They were undoubtedly the same disease, von Behring stated, insisting that *most* cases of pulmonary tuberculosis in childhood came from infected milk.

But Koch's opinion couldn't be dismissed. After all, his argument rested on his undisputed expertise with the microscope: Two different bacteria, he held, were responsible for the disease in the two host organisms. Almost immediately, governments in Britain, Germany, and the United States organized commissions to assess the evidence and reinvestigate whether there was, in fact, a link between the diseases.

The issue was more than merely academic. In recent years, public health officials in Europe and the United States had been recommending that all milk be purged of infectious microbes by a quick boil prior to sale. The process is known, of course, as pasteurization, after its inventor, and Koch's great rival, Louis Pasteur. Pasteur had created the method in the 1860s as a treatment for preserving wine, in order to rid it of uninvited yeasts. With a likely link between tuberculosis in humans and cows, it seemed natural to extend that process to milk.

Pasteur himself had died in 1895. It was somehow fitting that he would be coming back from the grave to confront Koch one last time. Even with one of them dead and buried, the two scientists were again on opposite sides of a debate.

Within a few months, the various commissions began to deliver their verdicts. Alas, it seemed clear that Koch was absolutely and outrageously wrong. The microbe, the American and British groups reported, was the same in both humans and cows; it was just that the tubercle bacilli, so wily all along, took a slightly different form in the bovine. (The German commission, misguidedly, sided with its national hero.) As von Behring had insisted, infected milk was a significant source of tuberculosis infection in humans. The statistics were unequivocal: In New York and Britain, as many as two-thirds of childhood cases were attributable to infected milk. Among adults, cases of crossover infection were less common, but they did, undoubtedly, happen often enough to be of great concern. The research convinced many cities, especially in the United States, to mandate the pasteurization of milk. Those cities that did so soon saw the number of TB cases drop significantly. Alas, in Europe, particularly in the United Kingdom, farmers resisted such measures, unnecessarily dooming many citizens to a fatal disease.

For Koch, it was a horrible blunder. He had once more stepped willfully into a controversy over tuberculosis. Once more he found himself squarely on the wrong side of the evidence. And once more he would refuse to concede his error. Though he had made his name on careful observation and meticulous research, he had now twice shot off an opinion, cloaking it in his authority rather than heeding his own methods of investigation and reinvestigation. And now he had twice been proven wrong.

The embarrassment grew later that year, in the fall of 1901, when von Behring, not Koch, was selected to receive the first Nobel Prize in physiology or medicine. The Nobel Prizes had been generating excitement in science circles for several years, ever since they had been spelled out in the last testament of Swedish industrialist Alfred Nobel. This was to be the year for the first prizes, with the announcement scheduled for December 10, the fifth anniversary of Nobel's death.

The choice of von Behring, in recognition of his work on the diphtheria antitoxin, offended Koch, and not just because von Behring had worked under Koch in Berlin. Koch felt slighted also because von Behring's work would have been impossible without Koch's. The very notion of immunology and antitoxins relied on the bacteriology that Koch had standardized. It was Koch who had laid the groundwork for modern medicine—Pasteur as well, to be sure, but he was dead, and the prize could go only to the living. And who among the living had done more for medical science than Robert Koch?

The determination that von Behring's one antitoxin therapy was more prizeworthy than Koch's years of microbial discoveries once again put Koch on the less celebrated side of bacteriology. Just as Pasteur's treatments for anthrax and rabies sometimes outshone Koch's detective work, here von Behring was receiving the laurels (nothing less than the highest medical honor ever created!) because he had cooked up a treatment, rather than the process that enabled it. And Koch no doubt heard that, when von Behring arrived in Stockholm to accept the prize, he took the stage and promised to use the prize money to prove that human and bovine TB were the same disease. Even worse, von Behring said he hoped to develop a vaccination for tuberculosis in cows and perhaps in humans, too.

Koch's offense would only grow when, in 1902, the second Nobel Prize for physiology or medicine went to Ronald Ross, for identifying the mosquito as the vector for malaria, and then again in 1903, when the Nobel was given to Niels Ryberg Finsen, for treatment of skin diseases. Then, in November 1904, the news appeared in *Science* and elsewhere that Koch would at last be recognized by the Nobel commission and had been chosen to receive that year's prize. But it was a cruel rumor; the reports were in error. Instead, the Russian physiologist Ivan Petrovich Pavlov was invited to Stockholm that December, in recognition for his work on reflexes.

Koch's work, it seemed, would go unrecognized. Had his failed remedy so tarnished all his previous contributions? Had that one failure—and what was science without failure?—undone his many triumphs: the work on anthrax, cholera, the postulates, the wound theory, and the discovery of tuberculosis bacteria, perpetrator of such misery, the greatest disease of the age?

A year later, in October 1905, at last Koch received a telegram from Stockholm informing him that he would indeed receive the Nobel Prize in medicine. This time it was official: The award was being given, the telegram said, for his work in 1882 identifying the bacteriological agent of the worst disease that humanity had ever known, tuberculosis. In his Nobel lecture on December 12, 1905, Koch reflected on the current state of tuberculosis research, noting the dramatic decrease in fatalities from the disease since the mid-1800s. He attributed this drop-off to several factors, including better housing and health among the lower classes and "improved knowledge of the risk of infection," which is to say, acceptance of the germ theory. He also praised the efforts at removing contagious tubercular patients from the general population and sending them to sanitariums, which both improved the health of tuberculars and reduced the spread of the disease. He allowed, however, that hospitalizing all these people would be "out of the question," given their sheer numbers.

"If we look back on what has happened in recent years in the fight against tuberculosis as wide-spread infectious disease, then we cannot help but gain the impression that quite an important beginning has been made," he concluded. "If the work goes on in this powerful way, then the victory must be won."

In Koch's last years, more committees and honors would come his way. The Institute for Infectious Diseases was officially renamed the Robert Koch Institute. He took more trips to foreign lands, accompanied always by Hedwig. Still, he would never shirk controversy. At the 1908 International Congress on Tuberculosis, in Washington, DC, he doubled down on his insistence that there was no connection between bovine and human tuberculosis. But this time, the reaction was rather cool. Where in previous years his opinion had forced international investigations and would have swayed his colleagues and steered the agenda, this time he was the outlier. In its final resolutions, the congress repeatedly contradicted Koch's conclusions, choosing instead to recognize bovine tuberculosis as contagious. As one delegate remarked, "Dr. Koch isolated the tubercle bacteria; today, science has isolated Dr. Koch."

Even in his moments of greatest glory, Koch was always the outsider. Science for him had begun as the pure pursuit of knowledge, and it was that focus, that purity of purpose, that allowed him to make his breakthroughs. His deep flaw was that, like so many men, he hungered not just for discovery, but also for the glory and recognition and stature that came with it. He overreached, and then he castigated those who would hold him to his own standards. He claimed a cure before he had the evidence, and then spent the rest of his life trying to prove his point.

In 1904, when he could plainly see the field of tuberculosis research drifting away from him, he wrote to a friend from his Breslau
days, who knew him when he was an unknown country physician and
who was there when bacteriologists seemed to have the gods at their
backs. "Your letter most vividly takes me back to the old days," Koch
wrote,

> when we could freely and without interference pursue our
> studies. Over time, this has greatly changed, alas. Whatever I
> tackle and undertake nowadays, a crowd of jealous and re-
> sentful individuals always turns up and jumps onto the same
> subject in order to start a controversy. . . . Today every little
> yapping dog will inoculate a single calf, write half a dozen
> articles about it afterward and carry on as if this case of his
> has solved the whole question, and of course in his favor. . . .
> Yes indeed, research would be a fine thing if everyone could
> think logically, but unfortunately this is the case for a small
> fraction only. Besides I believe that in my work my lot was
> particularly hard and I encountered more criticism, unjus-
> tified criticism, than anyone else.

Even in his last years, Koch couldn't quite admit that more than
any enemy or adversary, he was the agent of his own disappointments.

IN MARCH 1910, KOCH WAS BACK IN HIS LABORATORY IN BERLIN,
once again working on tuberculin, when he felt a sharp pain in his
chest. It was almost certainly a heart attack. After another episode in
April, he arranged to move to the clinic of Dr. Franz Dengler, outside
Baden-Baden. As it happened, Koch was now just across the Rhine
River from Alsace, the territory that Germany had seized forty years
before, after the Franco-Prussian War. The clinic had opened as a
sanitarium in 1890, built, in classic protocol, next to a hot springs in

the Black Forest. In his first days there Koch reported feeling better. Perhaps he would be able to return to Berlin soon. Perhaps he might even return to the laboratory. Then, on the evening of May 27, he stepped out onto his balcony, taking in the fresh air and the sun setting over a nearby park. Just before dinner, a friend stopped by to check in on him. He found Koch on the balcony, slumped in a chair, dead of a heart attack. He was sixty-seven years old.

In 1901, Arthur Conan Doyle did what he had vowed never to do: He brought Sherlock Holmes back to life.

In March of that year, Conan Doyle had gone on holiday with his friend Bertram Fletcher Robinson in Norfolk, in the East of England. As they toured the area, Robinson told Conan Doyle about his youth in Devon and of the legend of Richard Cabell, a seventeenth-century local man who was rumored to have sold his soul to the devil and who led a pack of hellhounds across the moor for years after his death. Conan Doyle was inspired by the tale and began sketching out a mystery, "a real Creeper," as he imagined it. Since every mystery needs a detective, he revived his own, in Sherlock Holmes. And in August 1901, the first installment of this new Holmes novel appeared in *The Strand*. This was *The Hound of the Baskervilles*.

Conan Doyle made clear that, technically, the story didn't mean that Holmes had returned from the dead. He set the story in 1889, *before* the standoff with Moriarty at Reichenbach Falls. But chronology notwithstanding, Holmes was back, and the public was overjoyed. In that first installment, *The Strand* sold thirty thousand more copies than usual, and the story was celebrated as Holmes's—and Conan Doyle's—return to form.

The final installment of *Baskervilles* appeared in April 1902. Within eighteen months *The Strand* would have another Holmes story for its readers, and this time Holmes was back for real. In "The Adventure of the Empty House," Holmes turns up one day at 221b Baker

Street to surprise Dr. Watson. He survived the fall at Reichenbach Falls, he tells his friend, and spent the past three years (it was a ten-year absence in real time) traveling in Florence, Tibet, the Middle East, and, finally, France. "I owe you many apologies, my dear Watson," Holmes explains, "but it was all-important that it should be thought I was dead, and it is quite certain that you would not have written so convincing an account of my unhappy end had you not yourself thought that it was true." This wasn't just Holmes speaking to Watson; this was Conan Doyle speaking to the entire world.

What made Conan Doyle change his mind and bring Sherlock Holmes back from the dead? First, in 1900 Conan Doyle had spent several months serving with the British army in South Africa, where the Boer War was under way. He reported for duty as a surgeon in the Royal Army Medical Corps, and just as Koch had during the Franco-Prussian War three decades earlier, he soon discovered how odious war could be. "You can find your way from Modder to Bloemfontein by the smell of dead horses," he wrote in his diary. The human toll affected him deeply, particularly after an epidemic of typhoid fever that broke out among British troops. Though he'd written about infectious disease in his Koch essays a decade before, the face-to-face ravages appalled Conan Doyle. "The outbreak was a terrible one," he noted. "We lived in the midst of death—and death in its vilest, filthiest form."

Then, in September 1901, the American actor William Gillette brought his play *Sherlock Holmes* from Broadway to London. The play, a mash-up of various Holmes plots, had run to a packed house for eight months in New York. Audiences loved Gillette's embodiment of the Holmes character, down to the bent briar pipe, the cape, the magnifying glass, and the deerstalker hat. The magnifying glass had of course appeared in Conan Doyle's stories; Gillette found the prop particularly well suited to the theater and brandished it with a flourish. The cape and hat were not Conan Doyle's invention, but rather had appeared in Paget's drawings. But the pipe was all Gillette's inspiration, as was the phrase he added to the script: "Elementary, my dear Watson." (The line never appears in a Conan Doyle story.)

On September 9, Conan Doyle attended the play's opening night at the Lyceum Theatre. Though he knew of the play's success in New York, it was quite another thing to watch the crowd thrill to Gillette's performance with his own eyes. After the final curtain, Conan Doyle stepped out of the audience to join Gillette onstage. The applause went on for many minutes, and Conan Doyle, standing next to the physical embodiment of his detective, took bow after bow. It was a thrilling moment, giving him a visceral, firsthand encounter with how deeply people adored Sherlock Holmes. "Sherlock is going to be a *record*," he wrote his brother about the play, "and beat Charley's Aunt"—*Charley's Aunt* being the most successful play ever staged in London theater at the time, running for a record 1,466 performances in the 1890s. Though *Sherlock* didn't quite beat that mark, it was indeed a smash for several years.

There was also the matter of Conan Doyle's wife, Touie, and her health. Consumption still racked her. It had been nearly a decade now since her diagnosis, and she'd likely been suffering from the disease for years longer. After the Conan Doyles returned from Davos in 1897, they had immediately started construction on Undershaw, a new estate in Surrey. Conan Doyle had heard the area described as an "English Switzerland," with good air ideal for Touie's health. He spared no expense in creating a large, airy house situated to capture plenty of sunshine. But the disease held fast. Like so many millions before, Touie never shook it. She and Conan Doyle took other palliative trips, including several months in Egypt and a spell back to Switzerland, but full recovery was elusive, and by 1900 she was considered, in the language of the day, an invalid.

Conan Doyle, meanwhile, felt in the prime of life. He was too honorable, and too adoring of Touie, to do her insult, but in 1897 he had found another love. Her name was Jean Leckie, and for the next decade she would become the great platonic love of his life. Always in the company of a family chaperone (his sister or mother, most often), Conan Doyle began bringing Jean on various trips across Europe. Touie, apparently, never knew; he was careful to ask his mother and sister to destroy any of his letters mentioning Jean, lest Touie find them. (Thankfully, they were less than diligent about this request, allowing us to read some of the correspondence.)

But by 1902 he was a man living somewhat publicly with two loves—one an invalid and one unrequited; one who had been his partner in the past and the other, he hoped, in his future. "This is a high & heaven-sent thing, this love of ours," Conan Doyle wrote to his mother about Jean, in February 1902. "It has kept my soul & my emotions alive."

In the wake of *Baskervilles* and the play, he must have realized that he could never really escape Holmes. The detective may have been his creation, but the whole culture, from America through Europe and most certainly in Britain, had been captivated by this curious character. It wasn't something Conan Doyle could ignore any longer. Perhaps there was more life in Sherlock Holmes after all.

The matter was decided in early 1903, a few months after the last installment of *Baskervilles*. Conan Doyle received a letter from the editor of *Collier's Weekly*, a popular American magazine. The editor made an offer that Conan Doyle couldn't refuse: thirteen stories for forty-five thousand dollars—more than a million dollars in today's currency. By postcard, Conan Doyle sent his reply: "Very well. A.C.D."

By June 1906, Touie was faring badly. She had lost a good deal of weight in recent months and began to suffer fits of delirium, then other symptoms, including paralysis on her left side. Conan Doyle entertained the thought that these "may be a mere passing weakness," but the physician in him knew the truth. The disease was in its final stages. Touie's body could no longer stand the ordeal. On July 4, 1906, he telegrammed his family: "She passed in peace."

It had been thirteen years since she was first diagnosed with tuberculosis. Then just thirty-six years old, she had made it to forty-nine. Conan Doyle would spend the next year in mourning, much of it in a true depression, as he cared for his two children, now ages seventeen and thirteen. On September 18, 1907, he married Jean Leckie in London.

Conan Doyle would no longer shy away from Sherlock Holmes. The detective was back in a new *Strand* series again in 1908. For the next two decades, he would make irregular appearances. The last story featuring him, "The Adventure of Shoscombe Old Place," was published in 1927, some forty years after *A Study in Scarlet*.

The public adored each appearance of the scientific detective, but Conan Doyle himself began to take a curious turn. This man who had spent years championing medical science, in both practice and pen, instead became a devout believer in spiritualism and superstition. In truth, he had had an interest in the occult since his years in Southsea, but after Touie's death he seemed drawn to séances and mysticism and all sorts of deeply unscientific hokum. By 1918 he was publicly championing spiritualism, a quasi-religion that put great stock in psychics as spirit mediums and in communication with the dead.

The public more or less politely ignored Conan Doyle's enthusiasms, happy to have the detective, whatever his creator might be doing. But it was impossible to ignore the spectacle that ensued in 1919, when photographs emerged of two girls from Yorkshire, Elsie Wright and Frances Griffiths, playing with fairies. About eight inches tall with ornate wings, and playing miniature pipes, the fairies appeared to be enjoying their time with the girls. Conan Doyle seized on the pictures and, in an essay published in December 1920 in *The Strand*, pronounced them real. After examining them with Holmesian techniques—"long and earnestly" with a high-powered lens—he declared that "these people are destined to become just as solid and real as the Eskimos."

The essay was a sensation, but the public was less than convinced.

"Is Conan Doyle Mad?" asked the *Daily Express*, dismissing the author's evangelism as "the ravings of a madman." Cartoons appeared mocking the author as a bewitched old man. But Conan Doyle stood firm: "I have learned never to ridicule any man's opinion," he responded, "however strange it may seem." Though fairy skeptics outweighed believers, it would be more than sixty years before the truth came out: The pictures were a hoax, the fairies mere cutouts from a children's book that the children gazed at while Elsie's father took photographs. "I thought it was a joke," Frances explained, "but everyone else kept it going."

Conan Doyle was once a great champion of science, one who had, through his great invention of Sherlock Holmes, helped convince so many millions of readers that science was a powerful force for good. And now he had been caught up in the most specious of fairy tales. His was an unfortunate delusion.

By Conan Doyle's later years, Sherlock Holmes was fast becoming the multimedia superhero that we know him to be today. Having already made the leap from books to theater, Holmes transcended another popular entertainment in 1929 when the first Sherlock Holmes talking motion picture, *Return of Sherlock Holmes*, came to London. In the audience was Arthur Conan Doyle, no doubt fascinated and tremendously impressed that this man he had cooked up half a century before in Southsea still held the public's attention. Conan Doyle died the next year, on July 7, 1930, of a heart attack.

Late in his life, Conan Doyle gave an address to the medical students at St. Mary's Hospital Medical School. Reflecting upon his career in medicine, such as it was, he offered what he considered medicine's greatest triumph. It was not any one discovery, Conan Doyle said, but rather the process of discovery itself.

In every literary or dramatic romance, you will observe that from the time that the villain is unmasked he is innocuous. It is the undiscovered villain who is formidable. So it has been in this wonderful romance of medicine. All this work of late years has been in the direction of exposing the villain. When once this is done, be he micrococcus or microbe, and be his accomplice a mosquito or a rat-flea, the forces of law and order can be turned upon him and he can be broken in to that human system which he has so long defied.

For Conan Doyle, the world of medicine and microbes was closely aligned to the world of law and order. Order out of chaos. Life out of death. Discovery out of obscurity. "And this part of the discovery," he suggested to the students, "lies with Koch." The address took place in September 1910, just a few months after Koch's death. Nearly twenty years after Conan Doyle exposed Koch's remedy as a false one, he still took time to admire the man's genius and to honor his legacy.

THE FIRST SHERLOCK HOLMES TALKIE THAT CONAN DOYLE EN-joyed in 1929 would stand on the threshold of a new era of enthusiasm for the detective. In the 1930s alone, more than a dozen movies featured him, including 1939's *Hound of the Baskervilles*. That film was the first to star Basil Rathbone, an actor who would go on to become associated with the character of Sherlock Holmes as strongly as William Gillette had been four decades earlier. (In all, since the first film in 1900, the character of Sherlock Holmes has appeared in more than 250 movies.)

In 1934 a group of devoted fans created the Baker Street Irregulars, a society that remains dedicated to the idea that Sherlock Holmes and Dr. Watson were real people and that, at most, Conan Doyle was a mere stenographer. Today, more than four hundred such societies are active worldwide, from Tokyo to Fort Meyers, Florida, to London. Indeed, Sherlockians were the original fanboys, embracing the characters and writing their own mysteries with them as early as the 1890s. Today, Conan Doyle's corpus of 56 Holmes stories and four novels pales next to the more than 3,400 stories in a dozen different languages that admirers have written and posted at fanfiction.net, an online bulletin board. (Conan Doyle's versions are better.) Though less than the number of fan-written Harry Potter stories, that's twice the number of *Vampire Diaries* stories. In London especially (though not surprisingly), the character is very much alive, with walking tours and pubs and monuments dedicated to him.

Some of this has devolved into kitsch, but the enthusiasm for Holmes—most of it, at least—remains true to the character that Conan Doyle created more than 130 years ago. In Holmes, we can watch science in action, not just for esoteric purposes but for the thrilling pursuit of criminals and mysteries. No matter what course Conan Doyle may have taken in his later years, in Holmes he created something that resonated with his age and all the years since.

Isaac Asimov wrote that Holmes was "the most successful fictional character of all time" because he represents the triumph of the "gifted amateur who could see clearly through a fog." Conan Doyle took what medical scientists a generation older than he—Joseph Bell, Lord Lister, and Robert Koch—had accomplished and mythologized their methods, turning their innovations into popular entertainment based on the singular principle that little observations can build into larger conclusions. Through Holmes, Conan Doyle helped people see how from a thousand small observations can come a profound and lasting change.

COMPARED TO ARTHUR CONAN DOYLE'S VIVID PRESENCE IN London, Robert Koch's legacy is rather inconspicuous in his adopted home of Berlin. He is a curious sort of artifact, one of those historical figures whose names appear on street signs and engraved onto building facades but are largely absent from public knowledge. There is, of course, the Robert Koch Institute, the great brick building on the banks of the Berlin-Spandau Ship Canal. Visitors there are greeted by an alabaster bust of the man, looking stern and tired, off to the side of the foyer. Down the hall, a small, well-kept museum is dedicated to his memory. There one can visit (by appointment) and see the microscope from Wöllstein, the stove Koch would incinerate his mice in after dissection, slides of his original tuberculosis cultures, and his handwritten notes for his first lecture on TB, from March 24, 1882. There is also a vial of liquid, translucent but dark brown, labeled "Tuberculin." At the end of the hall is Koch's mausoleum, an austere chamber, its walls lined with black-and-tan marble. On the checkered floor, beneath a profile of Koch etched into white marble, stands an urn filled with his ashes.

Curiously, there is a second Robert Koch museum in Berlin, this one located in the old Physiology Institute building, which was subsequently renamed the Robert Koch Forum. Here, in a small room down the hall from the library where Koch unveiled his discovery of the tubercle bacilli, are more microscopes, more bottles of tuberculin, and Koch's Nobel Prize and certificate. Visitors are infrequent, and with piles of papers stacked haphazardly in corners, it's as much storage room as museum. Near the Humboldt University of Berlin, where Koch once worked, there is also a Robert Koch Platz, a lonely square of grass with a massive granite sculpture of Koch wearing a long robe and looking off to his right. A small fence keeps anybody from stepping on the grass or getting too near the statue. The effect is oddly suited to Koch: The edifice looms large but the park doesn't have much purpose and is easily ignored.

That, aside from a plaque or two around Germany or Poland, or a lonely microscope displayed in the German Historical Museum, is Robert Koch's physical legacy. Where the names of Pasteur and Lister remain in circulation—Pasteur has his pasteurization and Lister has the mouthwash—Koch's name is most associated with the postulates, those abstruse dictates for how to pursue science.

As legacies go, the Koch postulates are rather abstract and out of date. The infectious process as Koch explained it became obsolete with the discovery of viruses, the mechanisms of which escape the net of his dictates. But the basic imperative behind the rules remains sound: *never B until A*. These postulates, and the process they speak to, are perhaps more enduring and beneficial to humanity than any one cure for any one disease might have been. That process is not a singular vaccine that can be injected or a pill to be swallowed; it is a now-pervasive concept, an enduring shift in the way people think. Koch perfected a method by which we could pursue science for the glory of discovery, for the purposes of knowledge, and for the betterment of us all.

It seems a perfect sort of poetry, then, that this man's greatest triumphs came because of his principles and that his most wretched failures came when he abandoned those principles. Before Koch, there was no succinct method by which to demonstrate causality, nor a recognized method to examine a treatment. In his postulates, he provided the former, and in his tuberculin trials, he provided the harsh inspiration for the latter.

Koch's contribution to science may not have been the cure he so badly yearned for, the remedy that tempted him into hubris. But he did create something. He convinced the world that germs existed and, in so doing, convinced the world that they could be defeated—if not by him, then by those who would follow.

The Cure

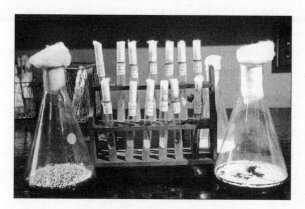

*Test tubes and flasks of the antibiotic streptomycin from
the Waksman Laboratory, circa 1945*

I t wasn't until the nadir of the Second World War—forty years after Robert Koch's death, fifty years after his supposed remedy, and fully sixty years after his initial discovery of *Mycobacterium tuberculosis*— when a true, real cure for tuberculosis would reveal itself, in the form of antibiotics.

This first agent to prove effective against TB was streptomycin, isolated by Albert Schatz, a graduate student at Rutgers University's College of Agriculture, in 1943. Under the direction of Selman Waksman, Schatz was exploring soil for microbes that might be turned into allies against other microbes. Though it seems odd to look in dirt for a germicide, on its face, there is logic to it. Just one gram of ordinary soil can contain billions of bacteria, many of which produce substances to ward off one another for competitive advantage. The great discovery of antibiotics was the realization that, by harnessing these inherent properties, bacteria could be turned into allies of humanity.

The approach had been validated years earlier, in 1928, when Alexander Fleming observed that a fungus, *Penicillium,* would naturally kill many kinds of bacteria. It would take more than a decade, not until 1942, before penicillin was purified into a dependable treatment for infectious diseases (among them staph, strep, gonorrhea, and syphilis). But with that proof established, the race was on to beat bacteria at their own game and recover chemical agents from soil that might serve as instruments to defend human health.

Penicillin and the other first antibiotics were a true godsend, arriving in time to be put to widespread use in World War II. But they weren't a cure-all; many microbe-borne diseases were unsusceptible to this early generation of antibiotics—most disappointingly, tuberculosis.

Schatz's new agent, however, had more success in disabling and killing the tuberculosis microbe. It slipped between the microbe's thick lipid walls and disabled the bacteria (precisely *why* it works is still not fully understood today). Waksman recognized the significance of Schatz's discovery immediately; he himself had been researching possible antibiotic agents for the previous decade. Within eighteen months, he'd recruited the Mayo Clinic to conduct clinical trials of streptomycin and arranged with the Merck Company to manufacture the drug. By 1945, it seemed promising that, at long last, there now existed an agent that could take on this most ruthless of killers.

But even as the laboratory evidence mounted, the researchers were wary of being too quick to claim victory. They were mindful of Koch's mistake and of those who had since exulted before they'd proven their case. They also realized that these previous disappointments meant the burden of proof was higher. "We feared that disbelief of the results would be expressed because of the many previous false hopes raised by other 'cures' throughout all previous medical history," said Horton Hinshaw, who was conducting the trials at Mayo. Nonetheless, the promise of the drug soon proved impossible to contain. The February 4, 1946, issue of *Life* magazine ran a lavish story devoted to the work of Waksman's laboratory, hailing streptomycin as "a new drug which is very much like penicillin but which cures diseases penicillin cannot." *Life* suggested that the drug's "greatest hope" would be in killing TB, which it noted worked in the lab but not yet in real trials. In most coverage, though, such subtleties were lost, and demand for the drug soon overwhelmed the Mayo team and anyone else involved with streptomycin.

Thankfully, this time the remedy did indeed work. On June 12, 1946, Hinshaw sent Waksman a telegram informing him of the completion of the first human clinical trials. "Our streptomycin studies . . . were fully confirmed experimentally and clinically, establishing this as first effective chemotherapeutic remedy for tuberculosis. Hearty congratulations." In 1952, Waksman would be awarded the Nobel Prize for the discovery of streptomycin; Schatz, unfortunately, would be deprived the glory of his discovery, as he was a mere student in Waksman's lab.

ALMOST IMMEDIATELY, IT WAS EVIDENT THAT THESE NEW "WONDER drugs" weren't without complications. Even in the first Mayo trials, some patients treated with streptomycin apparently recovered, only for the bacterium to return somehow, in a new form less vulnerable to the drug. This resistance was soon a regular problem with streptomycin, as it had been with penicillin, most gravely with staph infections.

The issue, it seemed, was that in some ways antibiotics worked *too* well, at least in terms of patient experience. The drugs quickly pushed the disease onto its heels, and patients would feel better within days and feel cured within weeks. But the bacteria were still there, hiding in the caseous material that the body had assembled to wall them off.

Now, though, that defense turned into a liability. Inside the body, the microbe was reproducing, with some generations of it creating genetic modifications that proved more resilient to the antibiotic. These new resistant microbes could remount their attack on the body, and additional rounds of streptomycin were ineffective.

The problem of resistance is one of simple math. A patient with extensive tuberculosis will have as many as one trillion bacterial cells in his body. Since microbes reproduce every few minutes or hours (tuberculosis reproduces at a rather languid fifteen- to twenty-hour cycle), there will be millions, or perhaps even billions, of opportunities for new generations of the bacterium to have slight mutations. Repeated over the course of weeks and months, the microbe might eventually find a path past a drug that may have worked just weeks before.

In the years after streptomycin was discovered, scientists were at first unworried about resistance, simply because so many other worthy antibiotics were emerging. With each one, humanity's newfound dominant role over disease seemed to be reinforced. These new drugs—isoniazid, rifampicin, pyrazinamide—worked even better in combination therapies, where a patient would take two drugs at once for several weeks or months. This protocol quickly became the standard treatment, since the odds that bacteria could successfully generate resistance to two drugs simultaneously seemed remote. Even when these new drugs began to show resistance as well, in the late 1950s, the combination could be altered enough to beat back the disease. Meanwhile, cases of tuberculosis dropped steadily in the United States and Europe and across the globe. Within a decade or two, it seemed a relic of a premodern age.

In the developed world, the general public lost any perception of tuberculosis as a true concern. The new antibiotics, combined with postwar hygiene and sanitation standards, entirely eliminated the disease from routine experience. Tuberculosis began to seem as dated as the words that had defined it a century earlier—*consumption, phthisis, scrofula.* Eventually, even the National and International Lung Associations, which had formed at the beginning of the century to combat TB, shifted their mission to another insidious threat to human health: cigarettes.

IN THE EARLY 1970S, THE US CENTERS FOR DISEASE CONTROL AND Prevention stopped direct funding of TB control, and Congress stopped requiring states to fund TB programs. Globally, the situation was similar, as the World Health Organization dismantled its TB program. There was little argument; the disease seemed like it was going away all on its own. In the United States, cases of tuberculosis had dipped below twenty-five thousand annually, compelling the CDC, in 1989, to release *A Strategic Plan for the Elimination of Tuberculosis in the United States.*

But the bacterium, unaware of humanity's inherent inconstancy, persevered and was well situated for the lapse in attention. Between 1985 and 1992, rates among adults soared by 20 percent, and among children, by 35 percent. The cause of the resurgence was tied largely to drug use among low-income populations and to HIV infections, which lower the body's resistance to other infections. But microbes know no class; when two Wall Street commodities traders were diagnosed with the disease in 1992, exchange officials required nearly three thousand employees to undergo testing.

Meanwhile, across the globe, new strains of tuberculosis were emerging that seemed more than just tenacious against antibiotics; they seemed downright impervious to them. These new superstrains resisted not just one but two or more antibiotics in the medicine chest. For the first time in decades, people with tuberculosis might receive a full course of treatment, yet still die—and at alarmingly high rates. As many as 80 percent died of this new form of TB, which became known as multi-drug-resistant TB, or MDR-TB.

The arrival of MDR-TB alarmed the global health community,

from the CDC to the WHO. Humanity suddenly seemed out-
matched in this cat-and-mouse game. The available drugs were divided into first-line, second-line, and third-line treatments, with the
WHO issuing strong and precise recommendations on which drugs
to take in combination and when. But as sensible as they were, these
rules ran headfirst into the problem of human behavior (as baffling an
adversary as germs ever were).

The fact of the matter was that taking TB drugs was (and remains) an ordeal. The drugs must be taken for at least six months,
long after a patient feels better. At five hundred milligrams, the pills
can be so large they are difficult to swallow. And uncomfortable side
effects, including rashes, headaches, and nausea, are common. The
result is that patients with TB often stop taking their pills once their
symptoms wane, unwittingly affording the bacteria that essential
second chance to mutate and regroup.

The arrival of MDR-TB called for a different strategy, one that
required a new discipline among patients. Taking a page from the
successful military-like campaign to eradicate smallpox, the WHO
created a protocol for delivering antibiotics: "directly observed therapy, short-course," or DOTS. The basic premise here is simple. A
health official or responsible community member must witness the
TB patient taking his or her medication, every day, for six months.
Every day, a knock on the door, and every day, swallowing the pill, for
at least six months or as long as it takes to return a clear blood test
(often eighteen months or two years). Getting such a program to
work, however, is onerous in countries that lack medical infrastructure or the political willingness to compel their citizens to follow such
strictures.

Still, for those willing to endure it, the DOTS therapy has good
odds of success, as high as a 95 percent cure rate. But inevitably, as
many as one-third of patients drop out, becoming unwitting allies to
the disease. Following the now-inevitable pattern, this created a new
strain of the bacterium: extensively drug-resistant, or XDR-TB,

which the WHO first classified in 2006 as TB resistant to the standard first-line and at least one second-line treatment. To have XDR-TB is to be almost without hope of a cure at all. One drug after another is tried (always in combination), in a course of highly toxic chemicals that goes on for as long as two years. Even after all that, as many as half of patients will not be cured. In some countries, such as those in Eastern Europe, rates of MDR-TB or XDR-TB are as high as 20 percent of all reported cases. For the first time in sixty years, people can once again come down with tuberculosis and have no chance of a cure.

Still, the science continues. On the last day of 2012, the US Food and Drug Administration approved bedaquiline, a new drug to fight against TB. Known commercially as Sirturo and manufactured by Johnson and Johnson, the drug is considered the first new therapy to be developed against TB in some forty years. It works by inhibiting an enzyme the microbe needs to replicate and spread throughout the body.

As promising as the drug is, it is being reserved strictly for patients with MDR-TB, and then only in combination with traditional antibiotics. The concern isn't so much that it won't work. Rather, it's that if it is used too much and stops working, there will be simply nothing else left on the shelf.

THERE IS ANOTHER CONSIDERATION, ONE THAT SHOULD ONCE AND for all compel us to rethink our supposed war against microbes (if the saga of antibiotics has not done so already). It is simply this: Yes, the classic infectious diseases such as tuberculosis and cholera and diphtheria have mostly vanished from our everyday experience. But the diseases that have replaced them and that now account for the majority of deaths in developed countries—heart disease and cancer, primarily—even these so-called noninfectious diseases may turn out to have an infectious component to them.

The clues have been accumulating for decades. As far back as 1976, the German virologist Harald zur Hausen observed that cervical cancer, then a major cause of cancer deaths among women, was largely associated with the human papillomavirus, or HPV. A vaccine against the virus was developed in 2006, allowing for a population-wide prevention campaign. (In 2008, Dr. zur Hausen won the Nobel Prize in medicine.) In the United States, rates of cervical cancer have fallen by 75 percent since the 1970s, but the disease continues to kill hundreds of thousands worldwide each year, an entirely preventable toll. Meanwhile, HPV is increasingly associated with throat and other cancers.

Some diseases once considered the result of human behavior and lifestyle also appear to be caused, in truth, by pathogens. In 1982, Australian scientists Barry Marshall and Robin Warren discovered *Helicobacter*, a microbe that was persistently present in patients with chronic gastritis and gastric ulcers. In an echo of the early days of the germ theory, experts in the field gave Marshall and Warren's discovery little credence; it seemed absurd that a bacterium could cause something so well associated with stress and human biology.

Frustrated with the naysayers, Marshall decided to prove his point. In a classic demonstration of self-experimentation, Marshall swallowed a vial of *Helicobacter* bacteria and promptly developed a nascent ulcer. A subsequent round of antibiotics cleared the condition. Other, more traditional research bore out his and Warren's hypothesis that ulcers were caused by *Helicobacter*. Yet it would be a decade before other scientists replicated their findings and changed the consensus opinion.

In 2005, Marshall and Warren would be recognized with the Nobel Prize. Their work was among the first to establish the significance of what is today known as the microbiome—the ecosystem of microbes in and on our bodies that may have a profound impact on our health, for good and for ill. Other diseases that are now believed to have at least some microbial association include Alzheimer's, asthma, dementia, diabetes, and as much as 20 percent of all cancers.

The research into the microbiome had perhaps its most profound demonstration, though, when the first convincing association between bacteria and heart disease emerged. Heart disease, of course, kills more people than any other condition worldwide, including 47 percent of Europeans; globally, it causes 30 percent of all fatalities. But nearly all research has gone to establish some sort of behavioral or environmental link (smoking, diet, exercise, stress, and so on down the list), with a smaller fraction of known genetic causes. Except in rare cases of acute infection, such as infectious endocarditis, microbes have been largely thought irrelevant.

But in 2013, at least one such association revealed itself, in the form of trimethylamine-N-oxide, or TMAO. TMAO isn't a microorganism itself; rather, it's a product created by bacteria when they digest lecithin, a fatty substance common in certain foods such as eggs, milk, and some nuts. In a study published in *The New England Journal of Medicine,* a team led by Cleveland Clinic's Stanley Hazen found that human subjects with the highest levels of TMAO in their blood had about twice the risk of having a heart attack, stroke, or death compared with those who had the lowest TMAO levels.

The association between microbes and human disease here is less straightforward than in the case of tuberculosis. In TB, the causal mechanism is fairly obvious: TB bacteria directly attack and injure human tissue. In Dr. Hazen's research on heart disease, though, the chain of argument requires a few more links. First the human has to eat a diet high in lecithin, then the gut bacteria must feed on the lecithin and generate a sufficient level of TMAO as waste, and then the TMAO must circulate in the body over time. Only then, the theory goes, does the actual damage happen, when TMAO allows cholesterol to get into artery walls and prevents the body from shedding extra cholesterol. Once there, the cholesterol accumulates in the blood vessels, causing atherosclerosis. This is a complicated histology from microbe to diseased tissue, and one that is a long way from being proven convincingly, let alone to a level of proof akin to Koch's postulates.

Nonetheless, this research is captivating and persuasive—and it gestures toward a new germ theory. This new germ theory would allow that direct connections between microbes and human health are less evident—or at least require more examination. It would grant that the dependencies and effects between microbe and humankind are more complicated and that new relationships will emerge.

This new germ theory is based on the growing awareness of a microbiome—those one trillion microorganisms that live in our guts and on our skin, a trillion organisms that unwittingly affect the larger organism that is the human body. The science of the microbiome—a concept that was first coined in 2000 but that has gained mainstream traction only since 2010 or so—is devoted to the possibility that these microbes play a far more nuanced role in human health than ever conceived, even more than the great microbiologists such as Koch and Pasteur may have imagined. Where Koch believed in the linearity of bacteriology (if the germ existed in the body, he believed, then the disease must also exist, and vice versa), this new science of microbiomics assumes that there are myriad influences and interactions at work. Some are directly causal, as with *Helicobacter* and gastritis. But others, as described in the TMAO research, are far more complicated and potentially more profound.

Teasing out the possibilities and implications of these more tentative associations will likely occupy the next century of scientists. This new generation of germ theorists will have to contend with the many microbes that exist in us but have yet to be identified. They will have to sort out the consequences of our overuse of antibiotics. And they will have to provide a more nuanced but still convincing argument against eradication: the increasingly discredited and potentially self-destructive notion that all germs are dangerous and must be eliminated (as if such a thing were even possible).

Like their predecessors in the nineteenth and twentieth centuries, this century's scientists must explain to a skeptical public why such a thing as germs matter, and why our understanding of these invisible beings demands to be reconsidered. If it remains necessary to learn what role they play in disease, it will also increasingly be essential to learn how they affect our health.

As any microbiologist or infectious disease expert will tell you, if we treat disease as a battle against microbes, we are destined to lose. The bacteria precede us. They outnumber us. And they will outlast us.

ACKNOWLEDGMENTS

This book wouldn't exist without *The New England Journal of Medicine*. On December 8, 2005, the journal ran a handful of essays on "medical detectives," including a tribute to Berton Roueché, a brilliant *New Yorker* reporter who, for several decades, spun urban outbreaks into gripping mysteries. When I was growing up, Roueché's stories were a favorite in our house, and my father, a physician and lifelong subscriber to *NEJM*, sent me the issue. In a note, he drew my attention as well to a brief essay by Howard Markel concerning a certain coincidence involving Robert Koch and Arthur Conan Doyle.

I filed away the issue and, five years later, realized that this historical footnote was in fact a book begging to be written. Though my father is not alive to read this book, I'm grateful that before he died at age ninety he was able to read the original proposal. Nor would I have been so inspired if Conan Doyle's detective stories weren't also family favorites, particularly beloved by my sister Cecilia in our youth. Cecie's work in public health and her death during a global health project inspired my own efforts in the field. I dedicate this book to both of their memories.

The library at the University of Minnesota (where my father taught medicine for forty years) contains a splendid Sherlock Holmes collection, and the staff there, including Timothy Johnson and Arvid Nelson, were generous with their time and counsel. Heide Tröllmich, the curator of the Robert Koch collection at the Robert Koch Institute in Berlin, likewise contributed her time and expertise. I am also indebted to Christoph Gradmann and Thomas D. Brock, whose scholarship on Koch has been indispensible to my own efforts. I wrote much of this book at the Community Library in Ketchum, Idaho, a splendid institution.

It's also essential to acknowledge the help I received from today's technologies. I thank Twitter for finding me Marco Kalz of the Open University of the Netherlands, who generously translated several of Koch's early letters. Likewise, only with the Internet would I have found Annelie Wendeberg, a microbiologist at the Helmholtz Institute for Environmental Research in Leipzig, Germany, whose keen read of my manuscript helped me skirt several errors. I am also glad for the existence of Google Books, without which I would've never discovered many significant sources and archival materials.

There have been crucial readers, beginning with Chris Calhoun, my agent and—more vitally—my friend. Steven Johnson, whose brilliant work has influenced my own, generously contributed a thorough read and crucial improvements. Conversations with Bill Wasik helped me navigate several challenges, and Alison Byrne Fields lent an eye as well. As always, my sister Laura contributed sage advice on medical matters. There were also the master readers I held in mind as my ideal audience: Mary Rose Goetz (who knows mysteries!), Sue Wright, and Lynda Chittenden.

At Gotham, Megan Newman has been an astute editor, and this book is the better for her efforts. Thanks also to Bill Shinker for recognizing the potential of this unusual story and how deep it might go. I'm proud to be in their house.

I'm grateful for support from my friends at the Robert Wood Johnson Foundation, especially Brian Quinn, Steve Downs, Paul Tarini, and John Lumpkin. Matt Mohebbi, my cofounder at Iodine, kindly tolerated my excursions into the nineteenth century as we build something for the twenty-first. Tom Neilssen and the team at the BrightSight Group have been brilliant at helping me spread these ideas to the public.

Finally: In many respects, I've been preparing to write this book—with its mix of literature and history and science—since 1986, the same year I met Whitney Wright, who remains my most significant discovery of all. All love and appreciation go to her and to our two boys, Rex and Buck, who fear neither needles nor germs.

NOTES

INTRODUCTION

ix **In train after train** William Thomas Stead, "Character Sketch: Robert Koch," *Review of Reviews* 2, no. 12 (Dec. 1890): 547–51.

x **In the last half** René Dubos and Jean Dubos, *The White Plague: Tuberculosis, Man, and Society,* 1st ed. (1952; repr. New Brunswick, NJ: Rutgers University Press, 1996), xiv–xvi.

x **So the consumptives came** Christopher Gradmann, *Laboratory Disease: Robert Koch's Medical Bacteriology* (Baltimore: Johns Hopkins University Press, 2009), 128.

x **the Berlin police department** Thomas Brock, *Robert Koch: A Life in Medicine and Bacteriology* (Washington, DC: American Society for Microbiology, 1999), 209.

x **"serious danger to the public health"** Arthur Conan Doyle, "Character Sketch, Dr Robert Koch," *Review of Reviews* 2, no. 12 (Dec. 1890): 547–59.

xi **In England, as many as** H. O. Lancaster, *Expectations of Life: A Study in the Demography, Statistics, and History of World Mortality* (New York: Springer, 1990), 360.

xi **In the United States** Barbara Bates, *Bargaining for Life: A Social History of Tuberculosis, 1876–1938* (Philadelphia: University of Pennsylvania Press, 1992), 1.

xi **a plurality of deaths** Jörg Vögele, *Urban Mortality Change in England and Germany, 1870–1913* (Liverpool, UK: Liverpool University Press, 1998), 144.

xii **In England circa 1870, twenty-two people** Figures published in *The Accountant* (London), July 16, 1904, 79.

xiii **Infant mortality in England** Samuel H. Preston and Michael R. Haines, *Fatal Years: Child Mortality in Late Nineteenth-Century America* (Princeton, NJ: Princeton University Press, 1991), Table 2.5.

xiii **"To the drowning man"** Philip Peter Jacobs, *Fake Consumption Cures* (New York: Metropolitan Life Insurance, 1913), 3.

xv **"When he clearly eyes"** John Tyndall, *Scientific Addresses* (New Haven, CT: Charles C. Chatfield and Co., 1870), 29.

xvi **"Gentlemen, this is no humbug"** Quoted in Roy Porter, *The Greatest Benefit to Mankind: A Medical History of Humanity* (New York: Norton, 1998), 367.

xvii **"If once tried"** Advertisement in *The Christian Messenger* (London), Jan. 1885, 66.

CHAPTER I

---

3 **When the young doctor** Brock, *Robert Koch,* 19.

7 **"It's going awful here"** Quoted in ibid.

8 **"The smell of dead bodies"** Robert Koch to Hermann Koch, Metz, Sept. 20, 1870, in *Deutsche Revue* 16, no. 2 (April 1891): 92. **At Metz** Geoffrey Wawro, *The Franco-Prussian War: The German Conquest of France in 1870–1871* (New York: Cambridge University Press, 2003), 186–87.

9 **the Germans suffered** Valery Havard, *Manual of Military Hygiene for the Military Services of the United States* (New York: William Wood and Co., 1917), 12.

9 **Delirium is common** George W. Fuller, "Typhoid Fever Death Rates in American Cities," *Public Health Papers and Reports* 27 (1901): 100–102.

9   **He pined for** Robert Koch to Hermann Koch, Metz, Sept. 29, 1870, in *Deutsche Revue* 16, no. 2 (April 1891): 93.

10 **The Germans deployed** Wawro, *Franco-Prussian War*, 57–59.

10 **"battle squirt"** Charles Alexander Gordon, *Lessons on Hygiene and Surgery from the Franco-Prussian War* (London: Bailliere, Tindall and Cox, 1873), 101.

10 **The real agent of destruction** Wawro, *Franco-Prussian War*, 53.

11 **"It was not an unfrequent sight"** Gordon, *Lessons on Hygiene*, 194.

12 **Still, despite such appalling** Matthew Smallman-Raynor and Andrew D. Cliff, "The Geographical Transmission of Smallpox in the Franco-Prussian War: Prisoner of War Camps and Their Impact upon Epidemic Diffusion Processes in the Civil Settlement System of Prussia, 1870–71," *Medical History* 46 (2002): 241–64.

13 **"this preparation"** Gordon, *Lessons on Hygiene*, 124.

13 **One couldn't have designed** Patrice Debré, *Louis Pasteur* (Baltimore: Johns Hopkins University Press, 1998), 266.

14 **a fatality rate** Fielding H. Garrison, *Notes on the History of Military Medicine* (Washington, DC: Association of Military Surgeons, 1922), 179.

14 **"In this war"** Gordon, *Lessons on Hygiene*, 197.

14 **Klebs was stationed** Gradmann, *Laboratory Disease*, 42.

14 **One afternoon** K. Codell Carter, *The Rise of Causal Concepts of Disease: Case Histories* (London: Ashgate Publishing, 2003), 95.

14 **"I found rod-shaped bodies"** Gradmann, *Laboratory Disease*, 43.

15 **"Does disease follow"** Brock, *Robert Koch*, 30.

16 **"I will never regret"** Robert Koch to Hermann Koch, Metz, Aug. 27, 1870, in *Deutsche Revue* 16, no. 2 (April 1891): 91.

16 **Robert Koch returned** Brock, *Robert Koch*, 19–20.

17 **"the most ingenious book"** Samuel Pepys, Diary, Jan. 21, 1665, http://www.pepys.info.

17 **"By the means of Telescopes"** Robert Hooke, *Micrographia: or, Some Physiological Descriptions of Minute Bodies Made by*

Magnifying Glasses. With Observations and Inquiries Thereupon (London: Royal Society, 1665).

18 **Van Leeuwenhoek improved upon** Porter, *Greatest Benefit*, 225.

19 **In a bit of verse** Hugo Erichsen, *Medical Rhymes* (St. Louis, MO: J. H. Chambers and Co., 1884), 84.

19 **By 1873, Koch's practice** Brock, *Robert Koch*, 24–26.

20 **"We shall soon perceive"** "Professor Rudolf Virchow," *Popular Science Monthly* 21, no. 46 (October 1882): 838.

21 **Virchow was his own** Paul de Kruif, *Microbe Hunters* (New York: Pocket Books, 1926), 140.

21 **"it is no longer necessary"** Rudolf Virchow, *Scientific Essays* (Stanford: Stanford University Press, 1971), 149.

21 **"before microscopic forms"** Quoted in Alfred S. Evans, *Causation and Disease: A Chronological Journey* (New York: Plenum Publishing, 1993), 14.

22 **In humans** John Bertram Andrews, *Anthrax as an Occupational Disease* (Washington, DC: Government Printing Office, 1917), 19–21.

23 **For farmers** Nicholas H. Bergman, *Bacillus Anthracis and Anthrax* (New York: Wiley, 2011), 1969–74.

23 **A French veterinarian** Andrews, *Anthrax*, 9.

23 **He may have treated** Ibid., 52.

23 **On April 12, 1874** Brock, *Robert Koch*, 31–32.

24 **"Whether they are"** Ibid., 30.

24 **"My heart says"** Ibid.

CHAPTER 2

27 **For an hour, then two** Brock, *Robert Koch*, 32.

27 **As Koch's experiments** Ibid., 321.

28 **"It was my job"** Ibid., 31.

30 **At the time, death in childbirth** Geoffrey Chamberlain, "British

Maternal Mortality in the 19th and Early 20th Centuries," *Journal of the Royal Society of Medicine* 99, no. 11 (Nov. 2006): 559–63.

30 Semmelweis monitored the two Porter, *Greatest Benefit*, 369–70.

31 "Where are these little beasts" Ibid., 372.

31 In 1877, Klebs was confident K. Codell Carter, "Koch's Postulates in Relation to the Work of Jacob Henle and Edwin Klebs," *Journal of Medical History* 29 (1985): 353–74.

32 As the scientific journal *La Presse* René Vallery-Radot, *The Life of Pasteur*, Vol. 1 (New York: McClure, Phillips and Co., 1902), 129.

33 Thomas Kuhn proposed Thomas S. Kuhn, *The Structure of Scientific Revolutions*, 4th ed. (Chicago: University of Chicago Press, 1962), 2–5.

34 "In investigating nature" Joseph Lister, "Edinburgh Graduation Address, 1876," excerpted in Rickman John Godlee, *Lord Lister* (London: Macmillan, 1918), 388.

35 Though the hygiene hypothesis Torsten Olszak et al., "Microbial Exposure During Early Life Has Persistent Effects on Natural Killer T Cell Function," *Science* 366, no. 6080 (April 27, 2012): 489–93.

36 "great ideas, like species" Stephen Jay Gould, "The Wheel of Fortune and the Wedge of Progress," *Natural History* 98 (March 1989): 14–22.

37 In Wöllstein, he was far removed Brock, *Robert Koch*, 36–37.

38 "In recent times, our knowledge" Ibid., 43.

38 "Honored Professor!" Ibid., 43–44.

39 The next morning Ibid., 44–45.

40 "My experiments were" Ibid., 45.

40 "This man has made" Julius Cohnheim, *Lectures of General Pathology* (London: New Sydenham Society, 1889), xiv.

41 Cohn's home was warm Brock, *Robert Koch*, 48.

42 "whole business" Ibid., 82.

43 "I see from your letter" Ibid., 81.

44 After the invention of photography Normand Overney and Gregor Overney, "The History of Photomicrography," March 2011, accessed July 16, 2012, http://www.microscopy-uk.org.uk/mag/artmar10/go-no-history-photomicro.html.

44 "true to nature" Brock, *Robert Koch*, 62.

44 He began to correspond Ibid.

45 "I am well aware" Ibid., 65.

45 but there was little experimental Gradmann, *Laboratory Disease*, 54–55.

45 In Parisian hospitals Greg Seltzer, "The American Ambulance in Paris, 1870–1871," MA thesis, University of North Carolina at Wilmington, 2009, 22–23.

46 Surgery manuals Thomas Bryant, *A Manual for the Practice of Surgery* (Philadelphia: Henry C. Lea's Son and Co., 1885), 67.

46 Though Klebs had clearly Gradmann, *Laboratory Disease*, 55.

47 The scientific method Terrie M. Romano, *Making Medicine Scientific* (Baltimore: Johns Hopkins University Press, 2003), 16.

48 "The various researchers" Felix Victor Birch-Hirschfeld, quoted in Gradmann, *Laboratory Disease*, 56.

49 This was evident in the title Koch's essay was also translated into English as *Investigations into the Etiology of Traumatic Infective Diseases*, as in an 1880 volume published in London by the New Sydenham Society.

49 "In order to prove" Robert Koch, *Etiology of Traumatic Infective Diseases* (London: New Sydenham Society, 1880), 22–27.

50 In these principles Ragnhild Munch, "On the Shoulders of Giants: Robert Koch," *Microbes and Infection* 5 (2003): 69–74.

51 He was now in regular Brock, *Robert Koch*, 84.

52 In early July 1880 Ibid., 88–89.

CHAPTER 3

53   **Pasteur took the post** Debré, *Pasteur*, 279–82.

54   **"If it is terrifying"** Vallery-Radot, *The Life of Pasteur*, 271.

55   **"Do you know why"** Debré, *Pasteur*, 300.

55   **"If by chance"** Ibid., 289.

56   **"I obey a call"** Louis Pasteur to University of Bonn, Jan. 18, 1871.
     Quoted in H. H. Mollaret, "Contribution to the Knowledge of
     Relations Between Koch and Pasteur," *Journal of the History of
     Science, Technology and Medicine* 20 (1983): 57–65.

57   **"each of my studies"** Debré, *Pasteur*, 24.

57   **"the Beer of Revenge"** Ian S. Hornsey, *Brewing* (Cambridge,
     UK: Royal Society of Chemistry, 1999), 7.

57   **"While politics with"** Arthur Goldhammer, "Grumpy," *London
     Review of Books* 17, no. 19 (Oct. 5, 1995): 26–27.

58   **Pasteur had come to the germ theory** Debré, *Pasteur*, 87.

59   **Pasteur's first theory** Ibid., 194.

59   **"Everything indicates"** Ibid., 258.

60   **In the 1860s, Joseph Lister** Ibid., 279.

62   **He got to work** Ibid., 307.

62   **"the original drop of blood"** Émile Duclaux, *Pasteur: The History
     of a Mind* (Philadelphia: W. B. Saunders and Co., 1920), 251.

62   **In a letter to Cohn** Robert Koch to Ferdinand Cohn, July 15,
     1877, in Brock, *Robert Koch*, 70.

63   **To solve the mystery** Debré, *Pasteur*, 316.

63   **"You must prevent"** Ibid., 318.

65   **The experiment took place** Ibid., 396.

66   **"Here it is!"** Ibid., 400.

67   **"We now possess"** Louis Pasteur, "Summary Report of the Ex-
     periments Conducted at Pouilly-le-Fort, Near Melun, on the
     Anthrax Vaccination," *Comptes rendus de l'Académie des Sciences*
     92 (June 13, 1881): 1378–83.

67 "It is always possible" Editorial, *British Medical Journal* 2, no.
    1076 (Aug. 13, 1881): 290.

68 "every land in which" *The Lancet* 1, no. 3022 (July 30, 1881): 184.

68 "not once only" *Popular Science Monthly* 20, no. 10 (Dec. 1881): 245.

69 "Though a hard worked" Joseph Lister, "On the Relation of
    Micro-Organisms to Disease," *Quarterly Journal of Microscopical
    Science* 21, no. 81 (Jan. 1881): 330.

69 Though Pasteur had the spotlight Brock, *Robert Koch*, 114–16.

70 In the weeks following Ibid., 103.

73 "Of these conclusions" Ibid., 171.

73 "The theory on the role" Mollaret, "Contribution to the
    Knowledge," 57–65.

74 "M. Koch is not liked" Robert M. Frank and Denise Wrot-
    nowska, *Correspondence of Pasteur and Thuillier* (Tuscaloosa: Uni-
    versity of Alabama Press, 1968), 111.

74 Pasteur himself kept silent Debré, *Pasteur*, 407–8.

75 "When I saw in the program" Brock, *Robert Koch*, 174.

75 Privately, meanwhile Ibid., 174.

76 "Concerning inoculation" Robert Koch, "On the Anthrax In-
    oculation," from K. Codell Carter, trans., *Essays of Robert Koch*
    (New York: Greenwood Press, 1987), 97–107.

77 "You ascribe to me errors" Debré, *Pasteur*, 408.

77 Many historians, understandably Mollaret, "Contribution to
    the Knowledge," 57–65.

79 "Why did you hide" Louis Pasteur to Robert Koch, Dec. 24,
    1882.

81 For Koch in particular Brock, *Robert Koch*, 90–92.

81 The disinfection paper Ibid., 106–8.

82 In Paris, meanwhile Ibid., 105–7.

83 As late as 1883 Debré, *Pasteur*, 257.

83 Pasteur himself boldly René Dubos, *Pasteur and Modern Science*
    (New York: Anchor Books, 1960), 224.

CHAPTER 4

85 On the brisk evening Brock, *Robert Koch*, 126–28.

87 Later, Loeffler recalled Ibid., 128.

87 "If the importance of a disease" Robert Koch, "On Tuberculosis," from Codell Carter, trans., *Essays of Robert Koch*, 83.

87 The usual technique Frank Ryan, *The Forgotten Plague: How the Battle Against Tuberculosis Was Won—and Lost* (Boston: Little, Brown and Co., 1993), 11–12.

88 There was no applause Brock, *Robert Koch*, 128–29.

89 Simply put, more people Francis Sheppard, *London, 1808–1870: The Infernal Wen* (Berkeley: University of California Press, 1971), 16.

89 HIV/AIDS has killed Centers for Disease Control and Prevention, accessed March 14, 2013, http://www.cdc.gov/nchs /fastats/lcod.htm.

89 Six waves of cholera Dhiman Barua and William B. Greenbough, eds., *Cholera* (New York: Plenum, 1992), 5–7.

90 Tuberculosis was altogether Dubos and Dubos, *The White Plague*, 2–6.

91 By the end of the century George Allen Herron, *Evidences of the Communicability of Consumption* (London: Longman, Green and Co., 1890), 107.

91 This toll was particularly John Mann, *A Contribution to the Medical Statistics of Life Assurance; with Hints on the Selection of Lives* (London: J. Masters, 1865), 40.

91 "There is a dread disease" Charles Dickens, *Nicholas Nickleby* (Oxford: Oxford University Press, 2008 reissue), 637–38.

92 "a disease so frequent" Thomas Young, *A Practical and Historical Treatise on Consumptive Diseases, Deduced from Original Observations, and Collected from Authors of All Ages* (London: B. R. Howlett, 1815), 20.

92 "Consumptive patients" Logan Clendening, ed., *Sourcebook of Medical History* (New York: Dover, 1962), 433.

92 Early symptoms Bates, *Bargaining for Life*, 17.

93 One can get a sense "List of Tuberculosis Cases," accessed July 5, 2013, http://en.wikipedia.org/wiki/List_of_tuberculosis_cases.

93 It infused the poetry Dubos and Dubos, *White Plague*, 58.

93 Working people typically Allison Aiello et al., *Against Disease: The Impact of Hygiene and Cleanliness on Health* (Washington, DC: Soap and Detergent Association, 2007), 3–6.

94 During the "Great Stink" David S. Barnes, *The Great Stink of Paris and the Nineteenth-Century Struggle Against Filth and Germs* (Baltimore: Johns Hopkins University Press, 2006), 55.

94 "Why do we expectorate?" J. J. Lawrence, "Is Spitting a Crime?" *Medical Brief: A Monthly Journal of Scientific Medicine* 25 (1897): 389.

94 They spit, as a matter Alfred Bunn, *Old England and New England, in a Series of Views Taken on the Spot*, Vol. 2 (London: Richard Bentley, 1853), 372.

95 An 1847 French A. F. Chomel, *Elements of General Pathology* (Boston: William Ticknor, 1847), 158.

95 "When we consider" C. Theodore Williams, "The Contagion of Phthisis," *British Medical Journal* 2 (Sept. 30, 1882): 618–21.

95 In each droplet Dubos and Dubos, *White Plague*, 8–15.

96 Today's epidemiologists Ian Nelson, *Infectious Disease Epidemiology* (Burlington, MA: Jones and Bartlett, 2012), 151–58.

98 This was the error Timothy Alborn, "Insurance Against Germ Theory: Commerce and Conservatism in Late-Victorian Medicine," *Bulletin of Medical History* 75 (2001): 406–55.

98 "If contagion had anything" Henry I. Bowditch, "Is Consumption Ever Contagious?" (Boston: David Clapp, 1864), 12.

99 "There is hardly any" Sidney Coupland, "Extract from a Lecture on Tubercule," *The Canadian Journal of Medical Science* 7 (1882): 113.

99 **The hereditary theory** Bruno Meinecke, *Consumption in Classical Antiquity* (New York: P. B. Hoeber, 1927), 383.

100 **"In developing certain"** James Ross, *The Graft Theory of Disease, Being an Application of Mr. Darwin's Hypothesis of Pangenesis to the Explanation of the Phenomena of the Zymotic Diseases* (London: J. and A. Churchill, 1872), 240.

101 **Among those who believed** Dubos and Dubos, *White Plague*, 96–97.

101 **Just as the taxonomy** Ibid., 69–72.

102 **Koch's discovery, though** Gradmann, *Laboratory Disease*, 14, 32.

103 **More than 150 years** Wesley William Spink, *Infectious Disease: Prevention and Treatment in the Nineteenth and Twentieth Centuries* (Minneapolis: University of Minnesota Press, 1978), 6–7.

103 **Budd, who practiced medicine** Dubos and Dubos, *White Plague*, 97.

104 **The most substantial predecessor** Selman Abraham Waksman, *The Conquest of Tuberculosis* (Berkeley: University of California Press, 1964), 84–85.

105 **In 1881, on the eve** Dubos and Dubos, *White Plague*, 252.

105 **"In science the credit"** Francis Darwin, "Francis Garlton, 1822–1911," *Eugenics Review* 6, no. 1 (April 1914).

105 **Given credit or not** Ryan, *Forgotten Plague*, 289.

106 **The term was coined** Robert K. Merton, "The Matthew Effect in Science," *Science* 159, no. 3810 (Jan. 5, 1968): 56–63.

106 **Rarely had medicine** Michael Worboys, "Tuberculosis, 1870–1890," in *Heredity and Infection: The History of Disease Transmission*, Jean-Paul Gaudilliere et al., eds. (New York: Routledge, 2001), 91–92.

107 **"To those old-standing"** Editors, *Medical Times and Gazette*, April 22, 1882, 411.

107 **"The rapid growth"** "Dr. Koch's Discovery," *New York Times*, May 7, 1882.

108 **In the months following** Brock, *Robert Koch*, 139.

111   **"Dr. Doyle begs to notify"** Andrew Lycett, *The Man Who Created Sherlock Holmes: The Life and Times of Sir Arthur Conan Doyle* (New York: Free Press, 2007), 92–93.

112   **"On my map"** Alvin E. Rodin and Jack D. Key, *Medical Casebook of Doctor Arthur Conan Doyle* (Malabar, FL: Robert E. Krieger Publishing Co., 1984), 35.

112   **Born in Edinburgh** Lycett, *Man Who Created*, 20–30.

113   **Physically, he was a** Arthur Conan Doyle to Mary Doyle, Southsea, Nov. 1883, in *Arthur Conan Doyle: A Life in Letters*, Daniel Stashower and John Lellenberg, eds. (New York: Penguin, 2007), 210.

114   **"Just a line"** Arthur Conan Doyle to Mary Doyle, Southsea, Feb. 1883, in Stashower and Lellenberg, eds., *Life in Letters*, 189.

115   **"The pathological importance"** *The Lancet* 3060 (April 22, 1882): 654.

115   **"the splendid series"** *British Medical Journal* 2, no. 1302 (Dec. 30, 1882).

115   **Throughout the summer** *The Lancet* 3068 (June 17, 1882): 840.

116   **"Had a man the power"** Arthur Conan Doyle, "Life and Death in the Blood," *Good Words* 24 (March 1883): 178–81.

117   **In 2000, two data scientists** E. Andrew Balas and Suzanne Boren, *Yearbook of Medical Informatics: Managing Clinical Knowledge for Health Care Improvement* (Stuttgart: Schattauer Verlagsgesellschaft, 2000).

118   **A report issued** William C. Richardson et al., *Crossing the Quality Chasm* (Washington, DC: Institute of Medicine, 2000), 1–8.

118   **This requires an idea** Everett M. Rogers, *Diffusion of Innovations*, 5th ed. (New York: Free Press, 1962), 32–35.

118   **Rogers developed his model** Ibid., 35.

120   **"the evidence that it is"** G. W. Bulman, "Are Bacilli Causes of Disease?" *The Westminster Review* 139 (1893): 503.

120 **Rogers called this** Rogers, *Diffusion of Innovations*, 306.

121 **"as nicely furnished"** Arthur Conan Doyle to Charlotte Drummond, Southsea, Dec. 1882 or Jan. 1883, in Stashower and Lellenberg, eds., *Life in Letters*, 183–84.

121 **"as they serve the double"** Arthur Conan Doyle to Mary Doyle, Southsea, May 1883, in Stashower and Lellenberg, eds., *Life in Letters*, 197.

121 **He wrote an article** Stashower and Lellenberg, eds., *Life in Letters*, 186.

121 **"When pestilence comes"** Arthur Conan Doyle, "The Lay of the Grasshopper," in ibid., 200.

122 **Even the royalty** Michael Worboys, *Spreading Germs: Disease Theories and Medical Practice in Britain, 1865–1900* (Cambridge: Cambridge University Press, 2000), 132.

122 **The 1862 International Exhibition** *International Exhibition Jury Directory* (London: George E. Eyre, 1862), 79.

122 **Hydrotherapy was in vogue** Porter, *Greatest Benefit*, 392.

123 **Despite these quacks** Ibid., 351.

123 **The Lancet and the BMJ** Ibid., 354.

124 **As Conan Doyle described** Arthur Conan Doyle, "The Romance of Medicine," in *Conan Doyle's Tales of Medical Humanism and Values*, Alvin E. Rodin and Jack D. Key, eds. (Malabar, FL: Krieger Publishing, 1992), 466.

124 **"These germs, they give us"** Joseph Bell, *Notes on Surgery for Nurses* (Edinburgh: Oliver and Boyd, 1887), 72. Bell's book is dedicated to Florence Nightingale, chief of the nursing staff.

124 **"His strong point"** Conan Doyle, *Memories and Adventures*, (Newcastle upon Tyne: Cambridge Scholars Publishing, 2009), 15.

125 **"Let me once get my footing"** Arthur Conan Doyle to Mary Doyle, Birmingham, March 1882, in Stashower and Lellenberg, eds., *Life in Letters*, 151–52.

126 **Many physicians were willing** Porter, *Greatest Benefit*, 317.

127 **Indeed, to live in London** William John Gordon, *The Horse-World of London* (London: Religious Tract Society, 1893), 113.

127 **The average life span** Eric Morris, "From Horse Power to Horsepower," *Access* 30 (Spring 2007): 2–9.

128 **"No doubt it will be said"** Charles Dickens, "Inhumane Humanity," *All the Year Round* 15, no. 360 (March 17, 1866): 238.

128 **"They took a number"** Frances Power Cobbe, "The Rights of Man and the Claims of Brutes," *Fraser's Magazine for Town and Country* 68, no. 407 (Nov. 1863): 588–89.

129 **In 1875, Cobbe founded** Nicolaas A. Rupke, *Vivisection in Historical Perspective* (London: Croom, Helm, 1987), 269–71.

129 **"Doctors are daily assuming"** Frances Power Cobbe, "The Medical Profession and Its Morality," *Modern Review* 2 (April 1881): 296.

130 **"Are we to be leeched"** Nadja Durbach, *Bodily Matters: The Anti-Vaccination Movement in England, 1853–1907* (Durham, NC: Duke University Press, 2005), 13.

130 **In London and other** London Society for the Abolition of Compulsory Vaccination, *The Vaccination Enquirer and Health Review* 4 (April 1882), 54.

131 **"vivisecting staffs of Koch and Pasteur"** Frances Power Cobbe, "The Cholera in Egypt," *Zoophilist* 3, no. 15 (Feb. 1, 1884): 220.

132 **On some level** Durbach, *Bodily Matters*, 7–11.

132 **Start with whooping cough** Centers for Disease Control and Prevention, "Pertussis Outbreaks," accessed July 30, 2012, http://www.cdc.gov/pertussis/outbreaks.html.

133 **In 2011 there were nearly** World Health Organization, *Weekly Epidemiological Record* 86, no. 49 (Dec. 2, 2011): 557–64.

133 **"We live in a society"** Carl Sagan, "Why We Need to Understand Science," *Parade*, September 10, 1989, 10.

134 **"has opened up"** Conan Doyle, "Life and Death in the Blood," 178.

135 **"For fear delicacy"** Arthur Conan Doyle, letter to editor, *Medical Times and Gazette*, June 16, 1883, 671.

135 **"The death rate varies"** Rodin and Key, *Medical Casebook*, 104.

136 **"Someone described our condition"** Rodin and Key, *Tales of Medical Humanism*, 465.

136 **"those magic letters"** Arthur Conan Doyle to Louisa Hawkins, Southsea, Feb. 1885, in Stashower and Lellenberg, eds., *Life in Letters*, 238.

137 **"His wife calls his attention"** Rodin and Key, *Medical Casebook*, 88–89.

137 **"that small square"** Arthur Conan Doyle to Mary Doyle, Southsea, July or Sept. 1885, in Stashower and Lellenberg, eds., *Life in Letters*, 243–44.

CHAPTER 6

139 **Every November** Sarah Freeman, *Isabella and Sam* (New York: Coward, McGann and Geoghegan, 1978), 178.

140 **"My poor 'Study'"** Stashower and Lellenberg, eds., *Life in Letters*, 247–48.

140 **"This is, I feel sure"** As quoted in Coulson Kernaham, "Personal Memories of Sherlock Holmes," *London Quarterly and Holborn Review* 159 (Oct. 1934): 449–60, reprinted in Harold Orel, ed., *Sir Arthur Conan Doyle: Interviews and Recollections* (New York: St. Martin's Press, 1991), 42.

140 **"We have read your story"** Stashower and Lellenberg, eds., *Life in Letters*, 247–48.

141 **"for the shock I had suffered"** Ibid., 240.

141 **"After ten years"** Arthur Conan Doyle, "My First Book," *McClure's* 3, no. 3 (Aug. 1894): 225.

141 **"a man may put"** Ibid., 227.

142 **The publishing industry was** "Science in the Nineteenth-Century Periodical Index," accessed Nov. 14, 2012, http://www.sciper.org/introduction.html.

142 **Some of these** Geoffrey Cantor and Sally Shuttleworth, eds., *Science Serialized: Representations of the Sciences in Nineteenth-Century Periodicals* (Cambridge, MA: MIT Press, 2004), 221.

142 **Typesetting, which** Melissa S. Van Vuuren, *Literary Research and the Victorian and Edwardian Ages, 1830–1910* (Lanham, MD: Scarecrow Press, 2011), 154.

143 **In 1871, some 2,500** Bernard Lightman, *Victorian Popularizers of Science* (Chicago: University of Chicago Press, 2007), 34.

144 **Conan Doyle had little firsthand** Russell Miller, *The Adventures of Arthur Conan Doyle: A Biography* (New York: St. Martin's, 2008), 120.

144 **"I had been reading"** Arthur Conan Doyle, "The True Story of Sherlock Holmes, *Westminster Gazette*, Dec. 13, 1900.

145 **"a little queer in his ideas"** Arthur Conan Doyle, *A Study in Scarlet* (New York: Harper and Bros., 1904), 6.

145 **"His zeal for certain"** Ibid., 15.

146 **"The man was a respectful"** Conan Doyle, *Memories*, 15–16.

146 **"How in the world"** Conan Doyle, *Scarlet*, 25.

147 **"Dr. Conan Doyle's education"** Joseph Bell, "Mr. Sherlock Holmes," introduction to *A Study in Scarlet*, 1892 edition.

147 **"It tinges the whole"** Rodin and Key, *Tales of Medical Humanism*, 458.

147 **"We have frequent cause"** Editors, *Popular Science Monthly* 36 (Dec. 1889): 264.

149 **"unpredictable new ideas"** Freeman Dyson, *The Sun, the Genome, and the Internet: Tools of Scientific Revolution* (Oxford: Oxford University Press, 2000), 13.

149 **"without which the whole"** Lightman, *Victorian Popularizers*, 4.

150 **These publications aimed** Alan Rauch, *Useful Knowledge: The Victorians, Morality, and the March of Intellect* (Durham, NC: Duke University Press, 2001); and William H. Brock, *Science for All: Studies in the History of Victorian Science and Education* (Aldershot, UK: Ashgate, 1996).

150   "From a drop of water" Conan Doyle, *Scarlet*, 19.

150   In 1839 the British naturalist Laura J. Snyder, "Sherlock Holmes: Scientific Detective," *Endeavor* 28, no. 3 (Sept. 2004): 104–8.

151   The bounty of words Jerry White, *London in the 19th Century* (London: Vintage Books, 2008), 323–43. See also "British Slang: Lower Class and Underworld," accessed Dec. 18, 2012, http://www.tlucretius.net/Sophie/Castle/victorian_slang.html.

151   The 1850s and '60s saw panic Jacqueline Banerjee, "How Safe Was Victorian London?" *The Victorian Web*, accessed Dec. 16, 2012, http://www.victorianweb.org/history/crime/banerjee1.html.

152   The Metropolitan Police "History of the Metropolitan Police," accessed Dec. 17, 2012, http://content.met.police.uk/Site/historypolicing.

152   In fact, crime may have Stephen Inwood, *City of Cities: The Birth of Modern London* (London: Pan Macmillan, 2007), 230.

152   "I've found it!" Conan Doyle, *Scarlet*, 9.

153   In France, Alphonse Bertillon Snyder, "Sherlock Holmes: Scientific Detective," 104–8.

153   "skin furrows of the hand" Ronald R. Thomas, *Detective Fiction and the Rise of Forensic Science* (Cambridge: Cambridge University Press, 1999), 226.

153   "There is no branch" Conan Doyle, *Scarlet*, 142.

154   "I had high hopes" Stashower and Lellenberg, eds., *Life in Letters*, 247.

154   "attracted some favourable" Conan Doyle, *Memories*, 53.

154   "we may then, I think" Arthur Conan Doyle to Charlotte Drummond, March 1888, Stashower and Lellenberg, eds., *Life in Letters*, 252.

155   it earned more than forty Conan Doyle, *Memories*, 53.

155   Conan Doyle dutifully Stashower and Lellenberg, eds., *Life in Letters*, 266.

155   "gave my patients a rest" Conan Doyle, *Memories*, 54.

155   The fee would be Miller, *Adventures*, 119–20.

155   For his part, Conan Doyle Lycett, *Man Who Created*, 160.

156   "Detection . . . is, or ought to be" Conan Doyle, *A Sign of Four* (New York: Harper and Bros., 1904), 151.

156   "all upon technical subjects" Ibid., 153.

156   "When you have eliminated" Ibid., 195.

156   "the excellence of its style" Advertisement, *The Athenaeum* 3033 (Feb. 14, 1891): 206.

156   "strength and sincerity" Miller, *Adventures*, 122.

156   "He said that He" Stashower and Lellenberg, eds., *Life in Letters*, 277.

157   "My life had been a pleasant one" Conan Doyle, *Memories*, 60.

157   But in November 1890 *British Medical Journal* 2, no. 1132 (Nov. 15, 1890).

158   "A great urge came upon me" Conan Doyle, *Memories*, 60–61.

CHAPTER 7

162   The most recent pandemic Barua and Greenbough, eds., *Cholera*, 12–14.

162   The major source Chas A. Cookson et al., *Further Correspondence Respecting the Cholera Epidemic in Egypt* (London: Harrison and Sons, 1883).

162   The Germans offered Koch Brock, *Robert Koch*, 141.

163   "Cholera has almost disappeared" Ibid., 151.

163   The French team, meanwhile Ibid., 153.

163   On the morning of Émile Roux to Louis Pasteur, Alexandria, Sept. 21, 1883, translated in *The Lancet*.

164   Koch, though, was not yet Brock, *Robert Koch*, 154–58.

164   "In all cases" Ibid., 161.

165   "WELCOME VICTORS!" Gradmann, *Laboratory Disease*, 194.

165   "Just as 13 years ago" Ibid., 195.

165   "In less than a decade" Brock, *Robert Koch*, 167.

165 "As far as we are concerned" Ibid., 183.

166 "Herr Koch has nothing" Ibid., 190.

167 "When he had travelled half the way" Dubos and Dubos, *White Plague*, 146.

168 Jean-Paul Marat practiced *Dietetic and Hygienic Gazette* 26, no. 7 (1910): 420.

168 leech usage soared Spink, *Infectious Diseases*, 13.

168 Some argued that playing Dubos and Dubos, *White Plague*, 137.

168 "It frequently produces" Ibid., 139.

168 "many regular visitors" R. E. A. Dorr, "Guide to Chicago," *Columbus and Columbia* (Philadelphia: Historical Publishing Co., 1892), 832.

168 "There has been neither pain" "Correspondence," *The American Lancet* 15, no. 4 (April 1891): 137.

169 "more beneficial in the treatment" Dubos and Dubos, *White Plague*, 140.

169 This enthusiasm, inevitably John Rayner, *Cod Liver Oil: Its Uses, Modes of Administration, Etc.* (New York: Rushton, Clark, and Co., 1849), 7–8.

169 "It is pure water" Daniel R. Barnett, "William Radam and the Microbe Killer," *North Texas Skeptic* 18, no. 1 (January 2004): 1–4.

171 Inside these facilities Bates, *Bargaining for Life*, 41.

171 "We have tried in vain" R. Harvey Reed, "The Climate of Our Homes, Public Buildings, and Railroad Coaches, a Leading Factor in the Production of the Annual Crop of Pulmonary Diseases," *The Sanitarian* 26, no. 259 (June 1891): 519.

172 "I firmly believe" Oliver Wendell Holmes, "Currents and Counter-Currents in Medical Science," *The Writings of Oliver Wendell Holmes* (New York: Houghton, Mifflin, 1892), 203.

172 By the summer of 1890 Gradmann, *Laboratory Disease*, 99.

173 "rather melts or wastes" Brock, *Robert Koch*, 200.

174 "in the 5th hour" Gradmann, *Laboratory Disease*, 122.

174 "the least reliable results" Ibid., 118.

174 **On August 3, 1890** Stefan H. E. Kaufmann, "Robert Koch's Highs and Lows in the Search for a Remedy for Tuberculosis," Nature Medicine: Special Web Focus: Tuberculosis (2000), accessed Oct. 13, 2011, http://www.nature.com/nm/focus/tb /historical_perspective.html.

175 **On the main platform** Winslow Anderson, "Correspondence: The International Congress," *Pacific Medical Journal* 33 (October 1890): 618–25.

175 **"In this imperfect world"** Ibid.

175 **"What has been achieved"** Robert Koch, "On Bacteriological Research," from Codell Carter, trans., *Essays of Robert Koch*, 179.

176 **"Dr. Koch was shrewd"** Anderson, "Correspondence: The International Congress," 621.

176 **"Dr. Koch's address"** "From Our Special Correspondent," *The Lancet* 2, no. 3493 (Aug. 9, 1890): 301.

177 **The politicians had pushed** Brock, *Robert Koch*, 203.

177 **"Koch, like all scientific men"** Editorial, *The Lancet* 2, no. 3509 (Nov. 29, 1890): 1169–71.

177 **"Indeed, apart from the fact"** "Dr. Koch's Investigations upon the Treatment of Tuberculosis," *The Lancet* 2, no. 3505 (Nov. 1, 1890): 932–33.

178 **"It was originally my intention"** Robert Koch, "A Further Communication on a Cure for Tuberculosis," *Medical News* 57, no. 20 (Nov. 15, 1890): 521–27.

179 **"I have purposely"** Donald S. Burke, "Of Postulates and Peccadilloes: Robert Koch and Vaccine (Tuberculin) Therapy for Tuberculosis," *Vaccine* 11, no. 8 (1993): 795–804.

179 **"He has given the world"** Gradmann, *Laboratory Disease*, 128.

180 **"the seed of a discovery"** Editors, "Koch's Discovery," *Medical News* 57, no. 20 (Nov. 15, 1890): 526.

180 **"as one greater than"** "Koch's Great Discovery," *New York Times*, Nov. 16, 1890, 1.

180 **Some desperate souls** Dubos and Dubos, *White Plague*, 148–52.

180 "He assured me" Conan Doyle, *Memories*, 62.

181 "simply not to be had" Ibid., 61–62.

183 **Conan Doyle turned toward** This episode was well told in a wonderful essay by Howard Markel, "The Medical Detectives," *New England Journal of Medicine* 355, no. 23 (2005): 2426–28.

183 "A long and grim array" Arthur Conan Doyle, "Dr. Koch and His Cure," *Review of Reviews* 2, no. 12 (Dec. 1890): 552–56.

184 "Great as is Koch's discovery" Arthur Conan Doyle, "The Consumption Cure," *Daily Telegraph*, Nov. 20, 1890, 3.

CHAPTER 8

189 **And so, every day** Conan Doyle, "Dr. Koch and His Cure," 552–56.

189 "There was no stopping" Gradmann, *Laboratory Disease*, 129.

190 **Charles Pratt lived in Minneapolis** Bates, *Bargaining for Life*, 38.

190 **From Paris, Pasteur** Brock, *Robert Koch*, 205.

190 "All the world rejoices" Burke, "Of Postulates," 800.

191 "according to the rule" William Thomas Stead, "Dr. Robert Koch: A Character Sketch," *Review of Reviews* 2, no. 12 (Dec. 1890): 547–51.

191 **The basic structure** Stephen R. Bown, *Scurvy* (New York: St. Martin's Griffin, 2005), 95–100.

192 "Let those who engage" W. Bruce Fye, "The Power of Clinical Trials and Guidelines, and the Challenge of Conflicts of Interest," *Journal of the American College of Cardiology* 41, no. 8 (2003): 1237.

192 "Randomize, always randomize!" Klim McPherson, "The Best and the Enemy of the Good: Randomised Controlled Trials, Uncertainty, and Assessing the Role of Patient Choice in Medical Decision Making," *Journal of Epidemiological Community Health* 48 (1994): 6–15.

193 **Koch appears to have** Burke, "Of Postulates," 800.

193 "Day after day" Ibid., 801.

193 **Each facility followed** Gradmann, *Laboratory Disease*, 139.

194   Even how to administer Burke, "Of Postulates," 796.

194   "Against a background" Gradmann, *Laboratory Disease*, 129.

194   In terms of patient response Ibid., 130–32.

195   "The effects . . . are simply" Brock, *Robert Koch*, 206.

195   On November 22 Ibid., 199.

196   He was keenly aware Gradmann, *Laboratory Disease*, 102.

196   A London paper reported "Koch and Tuberculosis," *The Chemist and Druggist* 37 (Dec. 6, 1890): 778–79.

196   By December, his institute Gradmann, *Laboratory Disease*, 104.

197   "thousands of medical men" Brock, *Robert Koch*, 202.

197   "the clinician finds himself" Gradmann, *Laboratory Disease*, 133.

197   "the unease that creeps" Ibid., 141.

198   By year's end Ibid., 128.

198   Of 242 patients Brock, *Robert Koch*, 210.

198   On January 7, 1891 Gradmann, *Laboratory Disease*, 136.

199   "My new remedy" Brock, *Robert Koch*, 211.

199   "You must know" Ibid., 233.

200   "It is a capital mistake" Arthur Conan Doyle, "A Scandal in Bohemia," *Adventures of Sherlock Holmes* (New York: Harper and Bros., 1892), 7.

201   "we are . . . assisting" Burke, "Of Postulates," 800.

201   "the present speaker allowed" Gradmann, *Laboratory Disease*, 146.

201   "When, six months ago" Nicholas Senn, *Away with Koch's Lymph!* (Chicago: R. R. McCabe and Co., 1891), 3.

202   "did not meet" Gradmann, *Laboratory Disease*, 149.

202   A German magazine Ibid., 152.

202   "He is the one man" Harold C. Ernst, *Koch's Treatment of Tuberculosis* (Boston: Damrell and Upham, 1891), 2.

203   "is always found" Edwin Chadwick, "Report on Sanitary Conditions," *Report from the Poor Law Commissioners on an Inquiry into the Sanitary Conditions of the Labouring Population of Great Britain* (London: W. Clowes and Sons, 1842), 369–72.

204 "A vast deal of the suffering" Florence Nightingale, *Notes on Hospitals,* 3rd ed. (London: Longman, Green, 1863), 8.

204 "What does 'contagion' mean?" Ibid., 6.

205 In the 1880s and '90s Andrew McClary, "Germs Are Everywhere: The Germ Threat as Seen in Magazine Articles, 1890–1920," *Journal of American Culture* 3 (1980): 33–46.

205 The New York City Board of Health Warren W. Hilditch, "A Bacteriological Study of Soiled Paper Money," *Popular Science Monthly* 73, no. 7 (August 1908): 157.

205 "although the reception" Nancy Tomes, *The Gospel of Germs: Men, Women, and the Microbe in American Life* (Cambridge, MA: Harvard University Press, 1999), 80.

206 "The man who hawks" Morris Gibbs, "The Anti-Spitting Association Again," *Modern Medicine and Bacteriological Review* 2, no. 4 (April 1893): 91.

206 "How necessary it is" J. M. Emmert, "Prevention of Tuberculosis," *Biennial Report of the Veterinary Surgeon of the State of Iowa* (Des Moines, IA: State Printer, 1885), 30.

206 "Le crachat" David S. Barnes, *The Making of a Social Disease: Tuberculosis in Nineteenth-Century France* (Berkeley: University of California Press, 1995), 83.

207 In 1892 the first organization Tomes, *Gospel of Germs,* 115.

207 Koch arrived and soon Brock, *Robert Koch,* 320.

208 A decade later . . . Biggs opened *1886–1914: Immigration, the Bateriological Revolution, and Hermann Biggs,* New York City Department of Public Health, accessed Jan. 10, 2013, http://www.nyc.gov/html/doh/downloads/pdf/bicentennial/historical-booklet-1886-1913.pdf.

208 "The knowledge we now have" Hermann Biggs, "To Rob Consumption of Its Terrors," *The Forum* 16 (1894): 758–67.

208 In New York, fatalities Barnes, *Social Disease,* 8.

209 "There must be no more" Brock, *Robert Koch,* 219.

209 "would be placed" Gradmann, *Laboratory Disease*, 104.

210 At the time, critics gossiped Brock, *Robert Koch*, 239–42.

CHAPTER 9

211 "I came back" Conan Doyle, *Memories*, 62.

212 "I am leaving Southsea" *Portsmouth Evening Mail*, Nov. 24, 1890.

212 "a gloomy, ominous reception" Stashower and Lellenberg, eds., *Life in Letters*, 283.

212 The couple quickly Arthur Conan Doyle to Mary Doyle, Vienna, Jan. 5, 1891, in ibid., 284.

212 His output was prodigious Lycett, *Man Who Created*, 172.

213 In London, the Conan Doyles Conan Doyle, *Memories*, 66.

213 And as Conan Doyle considered Stashower and Lellenberg, eds., *Life in Letters*, 293.

214 *The Strand* seemed the ideal Miller, *Adventures*, 133.

214 "There was no mistaking" Stashower and Lellenberg, eds., *Life in Letters*, 293.

214 "gratuitous and a waste" Miller, *Adventures*, 145–46.

215 As it happened, 1891 "Influenza," *Encyclopedia Britannica*, 11th ed. (Cambridge: University of Cambridge Press, 1911).

215 Conan Doyle was in Conan Doyle, *Memories*, 67.

215 "It was one of the great" Ibid.

216 "I can testify how great" Rodin and Key, *Tales of Medical Humanism*, 458.

216 "Whoever sets sail" *The Book Buyer* 9 (1892): 440.

216 Paget wasn't the first Miller, *Adventures*, 140.

217 "it has long been an axiom" "A Case of Identity," *Adventures of Sherlock Holmes* (New York: Harper and Brothers, 1892), 63.

217 "Ours would be remembered" "The Age of Science," *Nature* 42, no. 1092 (Oct. 2, 1890): 556–57.

218 "show that the public delights" H. G. Wells, "Popularising Science," *Nature* 50, no. 1291 (July 26, 1894): 301.

219 "read *The Memoirs*" Henry Edward Armstrong, *The Teaching of Scientific Method* (London: Macmillan and Co., 1910), 16.

219 Even the bacteriologists Arthur M. Silverstein, *Paul Ehrlich's Receptor Immunology: The Magnificent Obsession* (San Diego: Academic Press, 2002), 148. Also Rodin and Key, *Medical Casebook,* 296.

219 *Strand* editor George Newnes Miller, *Adventures,* 141.

220 On one such jaunt Arthur Conan Doyle to Mary Doyle, South Norwood, Jan. 6, 1892, in Stashower and Lellenberg, eds., *Life in Letters,* 304.

220 In October 1892 Miller, *Adventures,* 143.

220 "I think of slaying Holmes" Arthur Conan Doyle to Mary Doyle, South Norwood, Nov. 11, 1891, in Stashower and Lellenberg, eds., *Life in Letters,* 300.

221 "He still lives" Arthur Conan Doyle to Mary Doyle, South Norwood, Jan. 6, 1892, in Stashower and Lellenberg, eds., *Life in Letters,* 305.

221 In early 1892 Lycett, *Man Who Created,* 189.

221 He considered turning Miller, *Adventures,* 144–45.

221 The official purpose Ibid., 151.

221 "The torrent, swollen by" Arthur Conan Doyle, "The Truth About Sherlock Holmes," *Collier's,* Dec. 29, 1923. Reprinted in *The Complete Sherlock Holmes,* Vol. 2 (New York: Barnes and Noble Classics, 2003), 684.

222 "I am in the middle" Arthur Conan Doyle to Mary Doyle, South Norwood, April 6, 1893, in Stashower and Lellenberg, eds., *Life in Letters,* 319.

222 "Killed Holmes." Arthur Conan Doyle, Diary, "The Norwood Notebook," accessed Nov. 12, 2012, http://www.bestofsherlock .com/ref/200405christies.htm.

222 One day, when she couldn't Conan Doyle, *Memories,* 84–85.

223 **"He seemed to think"** Arthur Conan Doyle to Mary Doyle, London, Oct. 1893, in Stashower and Lellenberg, eds., *Life in Letters,* 322.

224 **"The organizer of half"** Arthur Conan Doyle, "The Final Problem," *The Complete Sherlock Holmes,* Vol. 2, 559.

224 **"What excuse"** *The Literary News* 15, no. 2 (March 1894): 75.

225 **For years afterward** Ron Miller, "Doyle vs. Holmes," PBS *Mystery!,* Jan. 2001, accessed Jan. 9, 2013, http://www.pbs.org /wgbh/mystery/essays/doylevholmes.html.

225 **"Ah, but I did it"** "The Story of Dr. Doyle's Life," *The Bookman* 2, no. 8 (May 1894): 50–51.

226 **"What an infernal microbe"** Miller, *Adventures,* 163.

CHAPTER 10

227 **"In Europe"** Brock, *Robert Koch,* 243.

228 **"At home"** Ibid., 237.

229 **"I should estimate the extent"** Robert Koch, "Address Before the British Congress on Tuberculosis," London, 1901, quoted in Allen K. Krause, "Essays on Tuberculosis," *Journal of the Outdoor Life* 15, no. 11 (Nov. 1918): 327.

230 **But Koch's opinion couldn't** Brock, *Robert Koch,* 254–55.

232 **And Koch no doubt heard** "Behring's Recent Announcement in Regard to Tuberculosis of Cattle," *Journal of Comparative Medicine* 23 (1902): 36.

232 **Then, in November 1904** The announcement simply stated, "It is reported that the Nobel prize for medicine will this year be awarded to Dr. Robert Koch." *Science* 20, no. 515 (Nov. 11, 1904): 652.

232 **"improved knowledge of the risk"** Robert Koch, "The Current State of the Struggle Against Tuberculosis," Nobel Lecture, Dec. 12, 1905, accessed June 30, 2012, http://www.nobelprize.org /nobel_prizes/medicine/laureates/1905/koch-lecture.html.

233 **"Dr. Koch isolated the"** Brock, *Robert Koch*, 283.

234 **"Your letter most vividly"** Gradmann, *Laboratory Disease*, 113.

234 **The clinic had opened** "Baden-Baden Facts," accessed Jan. 11, 2013, http://www.bad-bad.de/gesch/r_koch.htm.

235 **"a real Creeper"** Stashower and Lellenberg, eds., *Life in Letters*, 478.

236 **"I owe you many apologies"** "The Adventure of the Empty House," *The Return of Sherlock Holmes* (New York: W. R. Caldwell and Co., 1905), 13.

236 **"You can find your way"** Arthur Conan Doyle, Diary, May 1900, accessed Oct. 18, 2012, http://www.christies.com/LotFinder /LotDetailsPrintable.aspx?intObjectID=4290311.

236 **"The outbreak was a terrible"** Conan Doyle, *Memories*, 114.

236 **Then, in September 1901** Lycett, *Man Who Created*, 261.

237 **"Sherlock is going to be a *record*"** Stashower and Lellenberg, eds., *Life in Letters*, 481.

237 **After the Conan Doyles** Lycett, *Man Who Created*, 231.

238 **"This is a high"** Arthur Conan Doyle to Mary Doyle, Undershaw, Feb. 1902, in Stashower and Lellenberg, eds., *Life in Letters*, 490–91.

238 **By June 1906** Lycett, *Man Who Created*, 311.

238 **"She passed in peace"** Stashower and Lellenberg, eds., *Life in Letters*, 534.

239 **"these people are destined"** Arthur Conan Doyle, *The Coming of the Fairies* (New York: George H. Doran Co., 1922), 55.

240 **"Is Conan Doyle Mad?"** Stashower and Lellenberg, eds., *Life in Letters*, 682.

240 **"I thought it was a joke"** Miller, *Adventures*, 410.

240 **In the audience** Stashower and Lellenberg, eds., *Life in Letters*, 683.

240 **"In every literary or dramatic"** Rodin and Key, *Tales of Medical Humanism*, 467.

242 **"the most successful"** Issac Asimov, "Why I Love Sherlock Holmes," *Newsday Magazine*, Sept. 2, 1984.

245 This first agent to prove Ryan, *Forgotten Plague*, 122.

246 Schatz's new agent Ibid., 125.

246 "We feared that disbelief" Horton Hinshaw, "Historical Notes on Earliest Use of Streptomycin in Clinical Tuberculosis," *American Review of Tuberculosis* 70, no. 1 (1954): 9–14.

247 "a new drug which is very" "Streptomycin," *Life*, Feb. 4, 1946, 57–60.

247 "Our streptomycin studies" Frank Ryan, *Tuberculosis: The Greatest Story Never Told* (Bath, UK: Swift Publishers, 1992), 280–81.

248 The problem of resistance Hugo L. David, "Probability Distribution of Drug-Resistant Mutants in Unselected Populations of *Mycobacterium tuberculosis*," *Applied Microbiology* 20, no. 5 (Nov. 1970): 810–14.

249 In the early 1970s Lawrence Geiter, ed. *Ending Neglect: The Elimination of Tuberculosis in the United States* (Washington, DC: Institute of Medicine, 2000), 35–36.

249 Between 1985 and 1992, rates among adults Centers for Disease Control, "Tuberculosis Morbidity: United States, 1992," *Morbidity and Mortality Weekly Report* 42, no. 36 (Sept. 17, 1993): 696–97.

249 when two Wall Street commodities Thomas J. Lueck, "Two TB Cases Prompt Commodities Exchange to Require Testing," *New York Times*, July 23, 1992.

249 As many as 80 percent TB Alliance, "MDR-TB/XDR-TB," accessed July 28, 2013, http://www.tballiance.org/why/mdr-xdr.php.

250 Still, for those willing Robert M. Jasmer et al., "Tuberculosis Treatment Outcomes," *Respiratory and Critical Care Medicine* 170, no. 5 (Sept. 2004): 561–66.

251 In some countries TB Alliance, "MDR-TB/XDR-TB."

251 On the last day of 2012 "FDA News Release," Dec. 31, 2012, accessed July 24, 2013, http://www.fda.gov/NewsEvents/Newsroom/PressAnnouncements/ucm333695.htm.

252 **As far back as 1976** Franco Borruto and Marc De Ridder, eds., *HPV and Cervical Cancer: Achievements in Prevention and Future Prospects* (New York: Springer, 2012), 12–14.

252 **In 1982, Australian scientists** "Interview: Barry Marshall," Academy of Achievement, accessed July 18, 2013, http://www.achievement.org/autodoc/page/mar1int-1.

253 **Heart disease, of course, kills** Melanie Nichols et al., *European Cadiovascular Disease Statistics 2012* (Oxford: European Society of Cardiology, 2012), 10–12.

253 **But in 2013, at least one** W. H. Wilson Tang et al., "Intestinal Microbial Metabolism of Phosphatidylcholine and Cardiovascular Risk," *New England Journal of Medicine* 368 (April 25, 2013): 1575–84.

254 **The science of the microbiome** J. Lederberg and A. T. McCray, "'Ome Sweet 'Omics—A Genealogical Treasury of Words," *The Scientist* 15, no. 8 (2001).

INDEX